Long-Term Care in Canada

Status Quo No Option

Ann Silversides

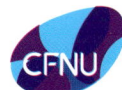

CFNU

CANADIAN
FEDERATION
OF NURSES
UNIONS

Published by
The Canadian Federation of Nurses Unions
www.cfnu.ca
2841 Riverside Drive
Ottawa, Ontario K1V 8X7
613-526-4661

This book was prepared by CFNU to provide information on a particular topic or topics. The views and opinions expressed within are solely those of the individuals to whom they are attributed, and do not necessarily reflect the policies or views of the CFNU, or its member organizations.

Project manager: Linda Silas
CFNU Researcher: Amanda Crupi
Advisory committee: Debbie Forward (NLNU); Beverly
    Mathers (ONA); Amber Alecxe (SUN)
Project team: Sean Dillon-Fordyce, Oxana Genina, Elizabeth Jefferson,
    Deanna MacArthur, Ismail Maniliho
Translation to French: Carole Aspiros

First Edition, February 2011

Library and Archives Canada Cataloguing in Publication

Silversides, Ann,
    Long term care in Canada : status quo no option / Ann Silversides.

Issued also in French under title: Les soins de longue durée au Canada.
ISBN 978-0-9784098-9-0

    1. Long-term care of the sick--Canada. I. Canadian Federation of Nurses Unions II. Title.

RA998.C3S45 2011   362.160971   C2011-900521-2

Printed and bound in Canada by
Imprimerie Plantagenet Printing   ®

FSC **Mixed Sources**
Product group from well-managed forests, controlled sources and recycled wood or fiber
www.fsc.org Cert no. SGS-COC-003420
© 1996 Forest Stewardship Council

Table of Contents

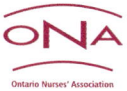

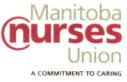

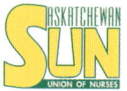

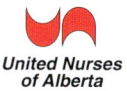

Newfoundland & Labrador
Nurses' Union

pei nurses
www.peina.com

Nova Scotia
Nurses
Union

NBNU SIINB

ONA
Ontario Nurses' Association

Manitoba
nurses
Union
A COMMITMENT TO CARING

SASKATCHEWAN
SUN
UNION OF NURSES

United Nurses
of Alberta

BC

CNSA·AEIC

Provincial Views

Continuing Care is an Essential Part of Medicare

A Champion of Medicare: Evelyn Shapiro

"I had a phone call from a landlady who rented an apartment to a woman who was 92 years old. She had been in hospital to have a cancer operation and had been sent home. The landlady visited and found that she hadn't eaten for 10 days. So we called the hospital and said, how could you send someone home like this? And we were told, well, the doctor thought she was doing very well and she could go home. Nobody thought to check to see if there was anybody at home. So when the Deputy Minister called me and said, are you ready to put your money where you mouth is, I went to work with the province..."

Evelyn Shapiro, 2007

Silversides, Ann. (2007).
Conversations with Champions of Medicare.
Ottawa: Canadian Federation of Nurses Unions. Retrieved from
http://www.nursesunions.ca/sites/default/files/Champions_inside1.pdf

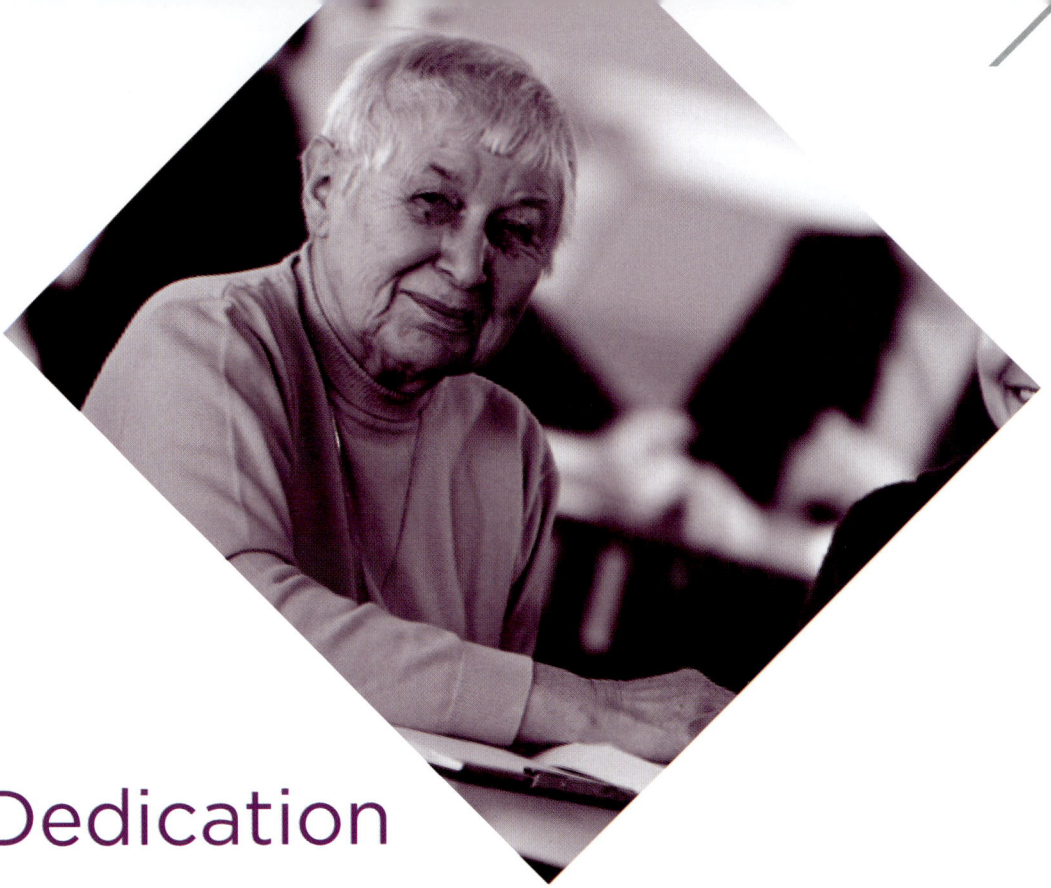

Dedication

This book is dedicated to Evelyn Shapiro who passed away while this book was being prepared for print. Evelyn Shapiro was widely known for her groundbreaking work in gerontology, home care, and related research. She was well known for developing and implementing the first provincial home care program in Manitoba and her research was instrumental in developing similar programs in other parts of Canada. Evelyn Shapiro was a recipient of many honours and awards, including an honorary Doctor of Laws degree from the University of Manitoba (2000), and the Order of Canada (2007). She was a passionate advocate for geriatric care in Canada and for medicare.

Message from CFNU
Linda Silas

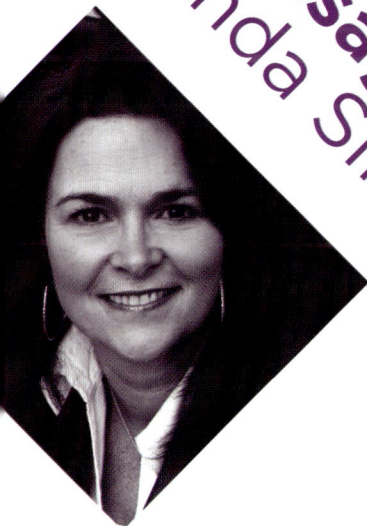

Dignity in aging should be afforded to every human being. It is the goal of many dedicated caregivers (formal and informal; paid and unpaid) to provide it to their clients, patients, residents, and loved ones. This project explores, from the perspective of national and provincial experts in long-term care, the challenges and realities facing the long-term care system in Canada, and the people who depend on it, including seniors and those with chronic illnesses. A common theme echoes throughout their stories: status quo is no longer an option for long-term care provision in Canada. The nature and needs of the population have shifted, but the system has not kept up. It is time we have a national discussion. It must also be realized that the need for change is urgent.

In 2009, the Canadian Senate released a report on Canada's aging population. Some of their findings paint a shameful portrait of how seniors in our country are living:

- Some seniors live in isolation or in inappropriate homes because of inadequate housing and transportation.

- Current income security measures for our poorest seniors are not meeting their basic needs.
- The current supports for caregivers are insufficient, and Canadians are forced to choose between keeping their jobs and caring for the ones they love.

The report also notes that Canada is facing challenges in health and social human resources — an issue all too familiar to our membership, as the introduction of skill mix models have drastically reduced the presence of nurses in long-term care facilities. In recent years, long-term care residents present with higher acuity rates and more co-morbid conditions — meaning that care plans can be complex and require a comprehensive approach to care. The stories within provide a strong message: set aside knee-jerk cost-cutting measures that do more to transfer rather than reduce costs. We cannot afford to undervalue the role of nurses in long-term care. There is no lack of research indicating that nursing care is strongly correlated to better patient outcomes as well as balanced budgets. What better way is there to honour our elders than providing them with the care they deserve?

The need for leadership and coordination through national strategies and initiatives that address the needs of patients and caregivers must become a priority for Canada. With 2014 fast approaching, discussions and negotiations are needed to realize the next *Health Accord*. These discussions must include pharmacare and continuing care strategies that specifically address long-term care needs.

The experts in this book provide us with a sense that a holistic approach to care is lacking in Canada and with this underlying message: where we fail to provide for basic needs — physical, social and cultural — we deny dignity.

Presently, the Veterans Ombudsman is undertaking a public consultation process on long-term care. The discussion on long-term care needs to be taken to the next level for the sake of all our seniors across Canada: a national consultation led by the federal government must accurately reflect the realities of our health care system, our health human resources, and our population's long-term care needs. There must also be an underlying understanding that the same principles that apply to health care in general also must apply to long-term care: access to quality care must not be based on means.

CFNU is one of many voices calling for action on long-term care: the Canadian Nurses Association, the Canadian Healthcare Association and the Canadian Union for

Public Employees are three other leading voices with expertise in this area, who share many of our concerns. It continues to be CFNU's mandate to work with health care stakeholders at every level and in every jurisdiction to create positive solutions to the challenges that face our nurses, our patients, and our health care system. We invite you to read this book and join us in a call to create a national discussion on this issue that must not be silenced any longer.

Linda Silas
President of the Canadian Federation of Nurses Unions

The Canadian Federation of Nurses Unions (CFNU) represents 176,000 nurses and student nurses in all provinces except Quebec. Our members work in hospitals, long-term care facilities, community health care, and our homes. CFNU speaks to all levels of government, other health care stakeholders and the public about evidence-based policy options to improve patient care, working conditions and our public health care system.

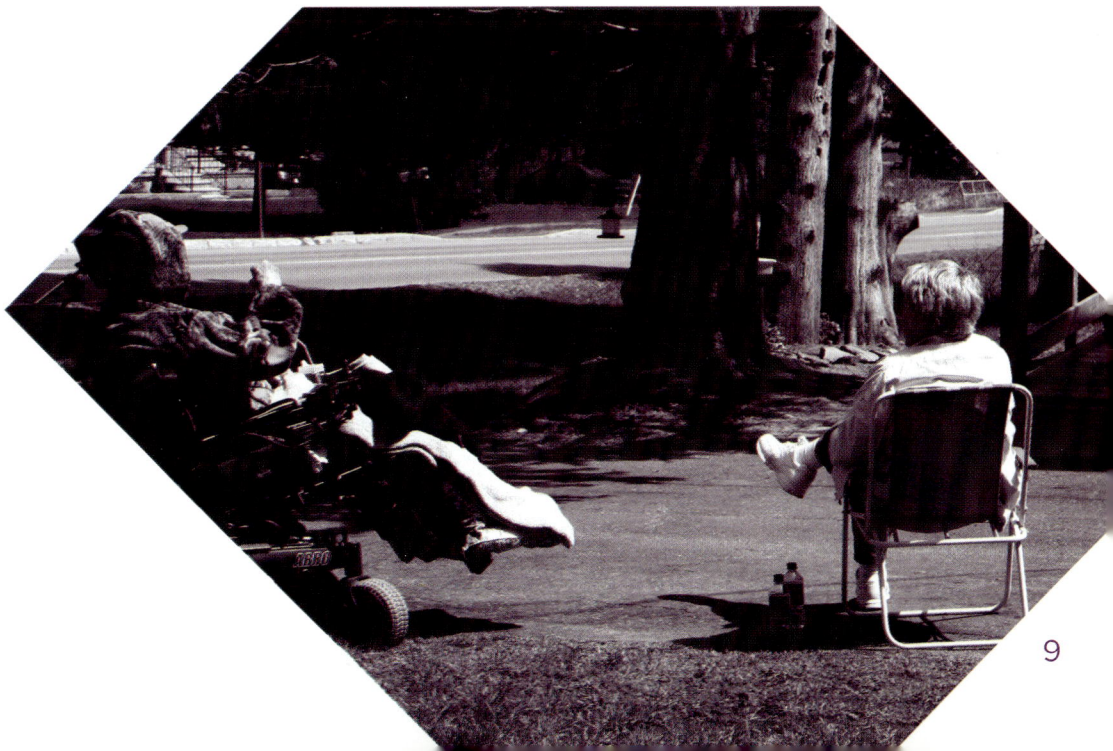

Residential Long-Term Care in Canada: Our Vision for Better Seniors' Care

This 2009 report on residential long-term care in Canada addresses two of the most urgent problems in the residential long-term care system: barriers to access and poor quality of care. The report also identifies what are thought to be two major driving factors underlying these issues: understaffing and privatization.

The Report's recommendations call on governments and employers to:

- Extend medicare to residential long-term care, with increased federal funding and legislated standards
- Expand home and community care services

- Phase out public funding to for-profit operators and end contracting out
- Increase staffing, with legislated quality of care standards
- Provide work environments that support high-quality care
- Support education and professional development
- Improve accountability and enforcement

In the report's press release, CUPE explains that "steady underfunding, understaffing and privatization have placed Canada's elderly in a two-tiered system where costs, access and quality vary depending on your income and where you live.

The solution — as outlined in the research — is increased federal funding tied to legislated standards of care, more care hours, and a phasing out of for-profit providers that cut corners at the expense of elderly residents."

Jansen, Irene. (October 2009). *Residential Long-Term Care in Canada: Our Vision for Better Seniors' Care.* Ottawa: Canadian Union of Public Employees. Retrieved from http://cupe.ca/elderly/report-seniors-care-crisis

Ann Silversides

Ann Silversides is an independent writer, editor and author. She spent more than 15 years as a reporter at the Calgary Herald, *the* Canadian Medical Association Journal *and the* Globe and Mail, *where she was the paper's first full-time health policy reporter. As a freelancer, she specializes in health policy and has written for a variety of publications, research institutes, unions and non-governmental organizations. In the 1990s she created numerous documentaries for the CBC Radio program* IDEAS *and in 2003 she published her book* AIDS Activist: Michael Lynch and the Politics of Community — *about the early days of AIDS in Canada and, for the Canadian Federation of Nurses Unions, she wrote* Conversations with Champions of Medicare *in 2007. Ann is the recipient of the Canadian Institutes for Health Research journalism award, the Atkinson Foundation fellowship in public policy journalism, and two Canada Council for the Arts awards.*

Introduction
Ann Silversides

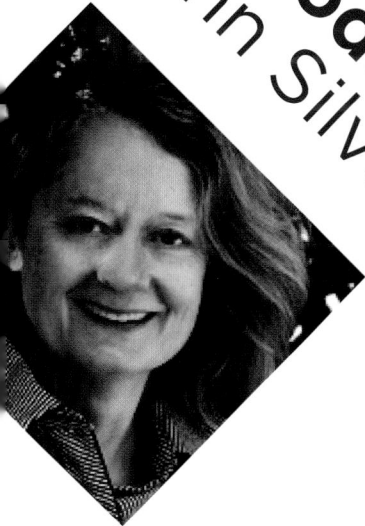

Home care services are being narrowed and cut. Nursing positions at residential long-term care facilities are being eliminated even though the medical needs of elderly women and men being admitted are much greater than a decade ago.

In the following pages, researchers, advocates and front-line workers from across Canada paint a disturbing picture. Their stories are red flags alerting us to a troublesome reality.

It unsettles me to realize that near the end of my parents' lives — my father died 28 years ago, my mother ten years later — the situation was actually better than now. More home care was available and a goodly proportion of residents in publicly subsidized long-term care were frail older citizens with minimal medical needs.

Today, instead of being well-funded and expanded so that aging Canadians can remain at home as long as they want, home care is mostly limited to medical care. Supportive home care that provides help with activities of daily living is almost non-existent.

When home is no longer an option, too many older citizens languish in hospital or pay for extra care while they wait for admission to long-term care facilities. After they are admitted to the facilities, inadequate staffing ratios often lead to neglect. Residents get diapers instead of help maintaining continence. Drugs are used to manage all sorts of behaviours.

"It physically hurts me to see what is happening; if these residents were people's children, there is no way they would be looked after this way. There would be an outcry about staffing ratios." That's how one nurse with years of experience in long-term care sees the situation. Another laments: "...we promised to provide the services to keep people at home, but we can't fulfil that promise."

Yet the issue of quality care for our elderly citizens is glaringly absent from election platforms and the national political agenda.

Across the country, there's a patchwork of services and accommodations for the elderly. Accessibility, cost, quality and staffing standards vary widely for both home and residential care. But there are commonalities, such as the increasing burden of the care that family members must assume whether their relative is at home or in a facility, the high rates of dementia and mental illness among those admitted to residential long-term care, and a significant increase in the number of drugs being prescribed for senior citizens.

My neighbours in the Ottawa Valley still live in the small lakeside bungalow they moved into 38 years ago. Margaret is 93 and sharp as a tack; at 82, Donny's memory and health are failing. A volunteer or a neighbour drives Margaret to town once a week for grocery shopping. Her son picks up their mail. When he can, he drives them to appointments. The couple is of modest means, and she is appalled at the cost of private retirement homes. They pay thousands of dollars a year for prescription drugs that are not covered by the public plan. Their doctor told me they should both be in the local nursing home, for which there is a one-year wait list. Right now, she wouldn't even be eligible and he wants to stay put: "The only way they will get me out of here is in a box." They don't qualify for home care.

In 2009, both the Canadian Union of Public Employees and the Canadian Healthcare Association published landmark reports: CUPE's *Residential Long-Term*

Care in Canada: Our Vision for Better Seniors' Care and CHA's *New Directions for Facility-Based Long Term Care,* and *Home Care in Canada: From the Margins to the Mainstream.*

These reports are rich sources of information; they draw attention to the urgent need to make improvements in the quality and accessibility of care for older Canadians. The two organizations come from different perspectives, so it is noteworthy that both are in solid agreement on the problems that now plague home care and long-term care, as well as many of the solutions. For instance, they agree that (in no particular order):

- understaffing in facilities is a huge problem,
- good work environments are essential to good quality care,
- quality of life (not just quality care) is vital,
- funding must be increased for both long-term care and home care,
- there must be an end to the exploitation of unpaid and informal caregivers,
- home care should not be pitted against institutional care,
- palliative care is underfunded in long-term care, and
- the care that is provided must be culturally competent.

The CUPE and the CHA reports are particularly comprehensive, but they build on and support the work of many other organizations and publications. These include the work of (among others) the Canadian, Ontario, and British Columbia Health Coalitions, the Canadian Centre for Policy Alternatives, the Consumers' Association of Canada, the Canadian Home Care Association, the Canadian Patient Safety Institute, and the jury recommendations from the 2005 Ontario inquest into nursing home deaths (the Casa Verde Inquest, formally known as the Inquest touching the death of Ezz-El-Dine El-Roubi and Pedro Lopez). As well, many academics and researchers, several of whom are featured in this publication, have devoted themselves to exploring ways to improve home and continuing care.

This book is complementary to the work noted above and, like it, aims to raise the profile of the care needs of older Canadians and to shine a light on the urgent need for improvements. The pages that follow feature the words of caring and compassionate front-line workers, advocates and researchers who speak from the head and from the heart. I hope it helps.

New Directions for Facility-Based Long Term Care

The Canadian Healthcare Association published a paper in 2009 which was considered a call to action on long-term care. The report aimed to raise awareness about the important role of long-term care homes in the lives of many Canadians. It lists a number of recommendations to all levels of government and stakeholders to address the challenges Canada faces:

1) Ensure adequate sustainable funding for facility-based long-term care tied to pan-Canadian principles
2) Focus on quality and accountability to Canadians
3) Invest in health human resources
4) Reflect a shared approach to risk
5) Guarantee reciprocity between the provinces and territories
6) Develop cultures of caring
7) Respect volunteers and families

Some key considerations include:

- Facility-based long-term care encompasses different services in each province and territory. It is not a publicly-insured service under the *Canada Health Act* nor a fully insured health service in any jurisdiction.
- There is a broad mix of public and private funding, ownership and administration of homes across Canada.
- Dementia and incontinence are the more likely conditions to necessitate admission to a long-term care home.
- In general, the non-senior disabled community and parents of children with disabilities do not favour placement in long-term care homes. Still, there are younger disabled persons often inappropriately colocated with confused elderly residents.
- Both accommodation rates and comfort allowances vary widely across Canada.
- The level of resident acuity and complexity of health services required in long-term care homes has increased dramatically since the start of the new millennium.

Canadian Healthcare Association. (2009).
New Directions for Facility-Based Long Term Care.
Ottawa: Author. Retrieved from:
http://www.cha.ca/documents/CHA_LTC_9-22-09_eng.pdf

Judith Shamian

Judith Shamian has earned many accolades and two honorary doctorates in her distinguished career in nursing leadership in Canada. She is currently the president and chief executive officer of the Victorian Order of Nurses, a 110-year-old organization that has played a pivotal role in nursing in Canada. Shamian has steered the VON through a period of significant transformation, bringing it under one organizational umbrella, and is working to secure its place as Canada's largest not-for-profit charitable home and community care provider through its next century of existence. She is championing the home and community care agenda in Canada, as well as working to strengthen partnerships between formal health care providers, families and friends who provide care, volunteers and community organizations in order to recognize and support the entire spectrum of care. Shamian, who has a PhD from Case Western Reserve University in Cleveland, Ohio, is in demand as a speaker and policy consultant nationally and internationally. She is a past president of the Registered Nurses Association of Ontario, past vice president of nursing at Mount Sinai Hospital in Toronto, and currently president of the Canadian Nurses Association.

National Experts
Judith Shamian

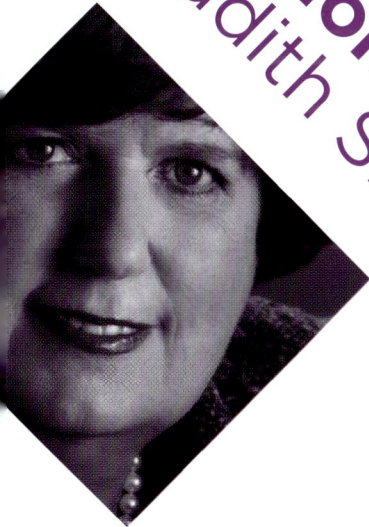

Chapter 1

What do you think are the key issues in continuing care for elderly Canadians?

First off, I am very interested in talking about integration of the system, and I think it is a risk philosophically to link home care to long-term care. Home care resides better with primary health care because home care does not take place in an institutionalized setting — the focus and locus of control is in the home and by the people who live there, whereas in hospitals and long-term care, residents have to fit into the organization's systems and policies. Also, I think there is an implicit assumption that if you can't manage at home, you have to go to a long-term care facility, and to me that is a flawed conversation. Let's say you can manage at home to a certain extent, but you can't shovel the driveway, or pick up your own medicine, or drive to see the doctor. If you build in community support — between voluntary organizations and other supports — then you can stay at home for another three to five years.

But surely it is not just families, volunteers and neighbours who should have to offer this home support?

No. And based on statistics, close to 50% of home care is now privately funded, through insurance or private money. That creates a discrepancy between those who can afford it and those who can't, and health shouldn't be a privilege, it should be something everyone is entitled to, despite the size of their wallet. We have funding for a program in Ontario in which the VON (Victorian Order of Nurses) has been given money to buy services to help elderly people at home. We do assessments and go out and source what they need in the community, not just from VON. And in the assessments that we have done — we used the standard instrument — our preliminary findings show that one third of people we support at home would normally be in long-term care facilities. There isn't sufficient appreciation that the solution for a lot of the problems in [demand for long-term care] and acute care resides in strengthening the home and community sector.

But there will always be people who need long-term care, correct?

Yes, and we need different layers of care. Some people will need ongoing clinical care and supervision, and then the question revolves around care from the regulated health professions, and what is the balance needed and what is the evidence. We do too much non-evidence-based care delivery. I would like to see more research and evidence in this whole area, so we could have solid policy advice, but research into care for the elderly gets crowded out by acute care and biomedical research. Meanwhile, the federal government has shown limited leadership, and there isn't enough pressure for solutions under the public not-for-profit system. The public needs to get urgently involved in this agenda.

What about support for family caregivers?

There is some data that 80% of care in the home is done by families. One of the things I am beginning to see in provinces is that they are starting to pay attention to how to support family caregivers — unpaid caregivers — and that is basically because they are beginning to understand that family caregivers are the main workforce. So when I talk about health human resources for the home and community sector, I talk about the challenges with the nursing and homemaker workforce, but in the same breath I talk about volunteers and family caregivers. Governments and businesses have to pay attention to the caregiver agenda — to offering flexible work time and other things. CEOs (chief executive officers) need to have policies that will support workers to be able to take care of families, so people can figure out how to take mom to see the doctor without standing on their heads or feeling guilty.

What was the impact of the introduction in 1996 of competitive bidding for home care services in Ontario? I understand that, as a result of the need to compete to provide home care services in a given geographic area, there has been a big increase in the proportion of care provided by large for-profit corporations.

It has been very traumatic to the sector and the people who work there, and it has basically been on ice [competitive bidding was halted] for five years, but it appears that it will get moving again soon. The cost of gearing up and writing proposals is phenomenal. We don't have enough funds in the system. By making home care a competitive industry in Ontario, there is little or no cooperation. It [The process] takes taxpayer money that could be used in different ways to support citizens in the system. We have done a comparative study between Ontario and Nova Scotia — the VON's two biggest markets for visiting and home making. We have hardly any staff turnover in Nova Scotia, where there is no competitive bidding and there is salary parity between hospitals and home care. But in Ontario, because of competitive bidding, there was a turnover of about 57% during the same period, and those who left have not stayed in the home care sector.

What is your prescription for the future?

One thing is that we need to build an awareness to understand that health starts at home, and to look at health in the broad sense — seniors staying active, seniors staying employed, seniors having a meaningful life past retirement. I think the baby boomers will put expectations and demands on the system, and I think we will build and encourage more community spirit and support. We will have to transfer the locus of control to individuals and families. It should be feasible to have a publicly supported system that approves the agency that you can use because it meets standards, and that provides you with some resources, so if four or five families choose to pool resources and hire and purchase care, they can structure it in such a way that the money goes further.

That sounds quite hopeful. What are your concerns about the future?

If we look forward to 2014 when the *Health Accord* expires, there are huge risks that the current federal government might not be eager to stay the course of funding, and if groups do not come in with some well thought-out strategies and push for it, it will be an easy target to use those dollars to help to balance the books. This is a huge risk for the whole health care system, not just home and community, but more so for home and community care since they are not part of the *Canada Health Act.*

Note: Following the 2003 First Ministers' Accord on Health Care Renewal, the federal government, in 2004, agreed to the 10-year Plan to Strengthen Health Care. Under the plan, the federal government agreed to transfer an additional $41.3 billion (on top of regular transfers) to the provinces and territories for health care improvements.

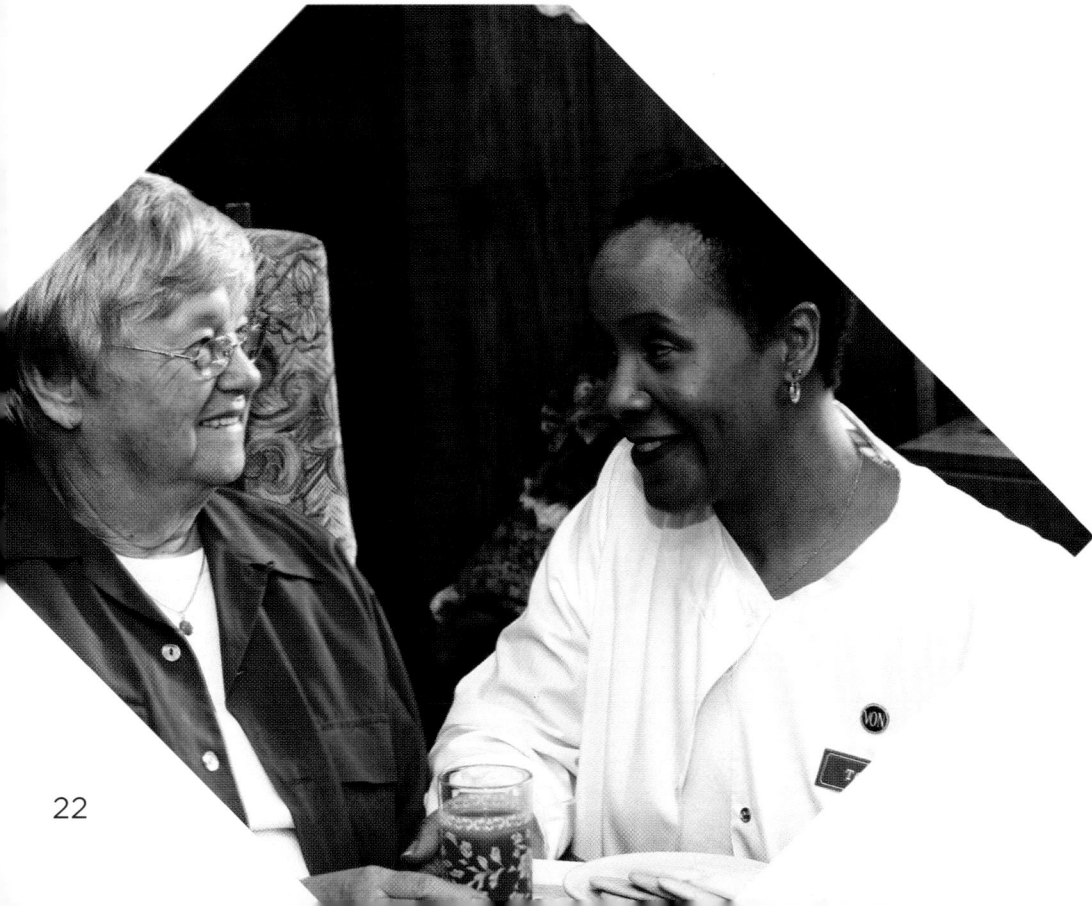

Domino Effect Caused by Lack of Access to Long-Term Care

"On any given day in Canada, alternate level of care (ALC) patients occupy the equivalent of approximately 7,550 beds in acute care hospitals. ALC refers to patients in acute care who are waiting for a transfer to a more appropriate setting, such as long-term care or a rehabilitation facility. In 2008–2009, there were more than 92,000 hospitalizations and more than 2.4 million hospital days involving ALC stays in Canada."

"When patients stay in acute care hospitals solely because they are waiting to be transferred to a more appropriate care setting, there is often a domino effect on the health care system," explains Murray T. Martin, President and CEO, Hamilton Health Sciences. "An acute care bed being used by someone who needs home care or long-term care is not available for a patient needing to be admitted from the emergency department, which may result in longer wait times for in-hospital admissions."

Canadian Institute for Health Information. (2010). *Health Care in Canada 2010: Evidence of progress, but care not always appropriate.* Retrieved from: http://www.cihi.ca/CIHI-ext-portal/internet/en/Document/health+system+performance/indicators/performance/RELEASE_16DEC10

Full report, *Health Care in Canada 2010,* can be accessed at: http://secure.cihi.ca/cihiweb/products/HCIC_2010_Web_e.pdf

Marlene Nosé

Marlene Nosé has extensive experience working with First Nations health organizations. She joined Health Canada in 1999, and is currently the Program Manager/National Coordinator of First Nations and Inuit Home and Community Care Program. Prior to joining the federal government, Nosé worked with First Nations health organizations coordinating, managing and integrating a broad range of community-based programs and services. Her early career also included extensive clinical experience in hospital and community settings such as public health, home care, and primary care. Nosé is a Registered Nurse with a Bachelor of Science degree in Nursing and a Master's degree in Public Administration with a concentration in health policy.

National Experts
Marlene Nosé

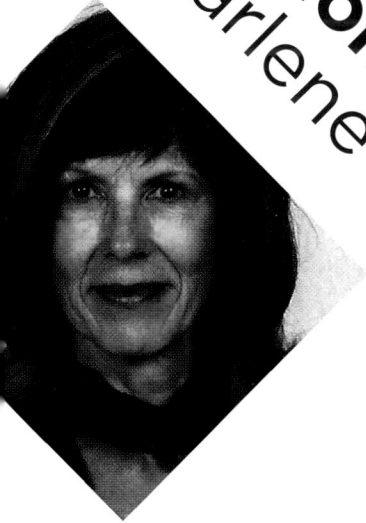

Chapter 2

What do you see as the key issues in the continuum of care for the elderly in First Nations and Inuit communities?

The issue now is filling in the gaps in the continuum of care. The main intent of our home and community care program is to keep people in their homes and communities safely, for as long as possible, and particularly to keep elders in the community so that they can participate in their communities and fulfil their role as elders. Our program [the First Nations and Inuit Home and Community Care Program] is 10 years old — people on reserves and in Inuit communities were not getting home care before 1999 — and now about 97% of the population has access to home care services.

So what are the gaps?

There are some clear gaps when clients are no longer able to stay at home and require high levels of care in an institutional care setting. Health Canada does not have the authority to deliver the higher levels of institutional care. INAC [Indian and Northern Affairs Canada], through its Assisted Living program, does fund lower levels of care, such as is provided at personal care homes or seniors lodges, and approximately 31 of the more than 600 reserves now have accommodation of this type. But many communities just don't have the population to support even these lower levels of institutional care. Also, facilities like seniors lodges are not licensed — or equipped or resourced — to provide higher-level nursing care, and provinces will only fund facilities on-reserve that are licensed. The other pressure point is palliative care, which is not one of our essential service elements, and nursing care services are not available on a daily basis.

What happens when people need higher levels of care?

Sometimes people who need more care refuse to leave their communities, but in most cases, people who cannot be cared for in their communities have to be moved to provincial care facilities. For example, in Ontario, people from Moose Factory are referred to Sudbury for higher-level long-term care, far away from their families and out of their cultural context. On the other hand, there is a provincially licensed long-term residence on the reserve on Manitoulin Island, and anyone in the community in that area can go there. However the Manitoulin situation is not commonplace.

It seems there are two complexities: the care issues, with 40% of First Nations over 60 having at least four medical conditions, and the complexity of the care system.

Yes, and we need to support better integration of our services with provincial systems so there can be a smooth transition. Now it is quite bumpy. A lot of work has been done in some provinces, but keeping good relationships with hospital discharge staff is an ongoing issue. I hear a lot about issues around discharge planning and referrals of clients from provincial institutions into the First Nations care delivery systems. We still have snags. A lot of work needs to happen at the First Nations organizational level to develop strong linkages with hospitals, doctors, other agencies and organizations, and that takes a lot of effort to maintain on an ongoing basis. It is difficult. Home care staff are so busy trying to meet needs at the community level that it is difficult to find time to hold meetings to develop and maintain effective linkages.

How have things changed over the last ten years?

In the early days of the 1990s, when our program was being set up, people were thinking more about responding to the rising rates of chronic diseases, especially diabetes, and caring for the frail elderly. They did not anticipate the impact of early provincial/territorial hospital discharge policies; our program was not designed to accommodate that. And while provinces and territories got money in the 2004 Health Accord to provide palliative, post-acute and mental health home care services, no increases were provided to First Nations and Inuit Home and Community Care Program at that time. What we see now is an increase in people who require a lot of intensive acute care and support [because of early hospital discharge]. And the ever increasing rate of chronic diseases continues to be a challenge for the program.

How do you coordinate with services offered by Indian and Northern Affairs?

Our services in the home are complementary. We provide home-based nursing and personal care — transferring, bathing and so on based on assessed need. INAC provides home support/home making services like cleaning and meal preparation. That's the difference. First Nations can offer more home-support services, that is where we have a bit of an advantage, whereas in provinces, unless you have a medical need, you don't receive home support, or you have to pay for it. But I should note that the INAC program is for First Nations only and does not include Inuit. Our program covers Inuit and First Nations.

What does the evidence say?

The burden on family caregivers is huge. The majority of home care is provided by families, and with early hospital discharge and the demand for palliative care, that burden is quite large. Respite care is one of our core elements, but data show some decreases [in the provision of respite care] over time, which tells me there isn't enough staff to go around to do the respite care that is needed. We are told the older population will double, at least, and greater demands will be placed on home care in the future. We have an electronic data collection system but we don't collect data on care that can't be provided, and that is one of the limitations of the system. But our continuing care research has documented gaps in the continuum of care — particularly higher-level care needs and palliative care. The rising rate of chronic diseases also presents challenges to the program.

What are your human resource challenges?

There are always issues related to the recruitment and retention of health care staff. It is an ongoing issue to hire and retain nurses and to have better systems to support nurses to work in communities. A lot of work has been done federally with the Aboriginal Health Human Resource strategy to support the development of more culturally suitable programs in universities and community colleges thereby improving access by First Nations and Inuit. In the home care programs many communities are now hiring LPNs (licensed practical nurses). We played a role in the beginning [of our program] to help training opportunities reach communities since our personal care workers have to be certified according to provincial/territorial standards. Improvements were also made to access LPN training. However, retention is an ongoing issue, and we find that once people are trained and certified, some of them choose to work in nearby long-term care facilities, or for home care agencies in neighbouring communities. This is an ongoing challenge.

What would you like to see in the future?

More resources and better partnerships and integration with provincial services. I think for the next ten years there will be terrific demands on the home care system. Right now the number one referral to our program is for clients with diabetes, followed by musculoskeletal conditions and heart and cardiovascular diseases. We currently do not know the number of people with Alzheimer's and dementia. However, I can see the future in terms of more issues related to Alzheimer's, dementia and neurological disorders. This will be a pressure point that will lead to the need for more respite care and will create more pressure for more institutional care settings. After all, there comes a point for many families where they just cannot manage someone seriously ill in their home — despite having support from a home care program.

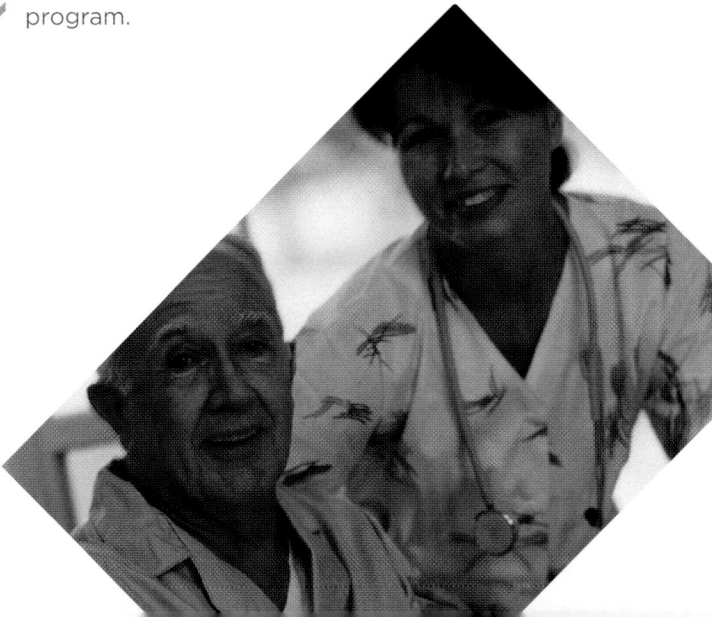

Continuing Care in First Nations and Inuit Communities

In 2004, the Government of Canada, First Nations and Inuit organizations undertook research into existing home and facility-based continuing care services in First Nations and Inuit communities. The report identified that:

- Families and caregivers require better access to home and community care during evenings and weekends and to respite care.
- The formal system should be structured to support families when they can provide the care. This is critical for families to manage their heavy loads.
- Continuing care services need to be designed so that they also address the higher care needs including long-term and short-term facility-based care.
- Supportive housing can also fill some of the gaps at lower levels of care.
- Various funding issues need to be addressed to meet the increased demand and higher level care needs and take into account case mix, community size and location and other factors such as culture and language requirements of the client, family and community.

Health Canada. (2007). *Continuing Care in First Nations and Inuit Communities: Evidence from the Research.* Ottawa: Author. Retrieved from: http://www.hc-sc.gc.ca/fniah-spnia/pubs/services/_home-domicile/2007_info_contin_care-soins/index-eng.php

Pat Armstrong

Pat Armstrong is a leading expert on the Canadian health care system and has co-authored or edited more than a dozen books on health care, including They Deserve Better: The long-term care experience in Canada and Scandinavia, Wasting Away: the Undermining of Canadian Health Care, *and* Caring For/Caring About: Women, Home Care and Unpaid Caregiving. *Now a sociology professor at York University in Toronto, Armstrong was formerly Director of the School of Canadian Studies at Carleton University in Ottawa. She is the Chair of Women and Health Care Reform — a working group of the Centres for Excellence for Women's Health, and holds a Canadian Health Services Research Foundation/Canadian Institutes of Health Research chair in health services and nursing research. Armstrong's current research projects include an examination of the risks nurses face in health care and a large collaborative project titled Re-imagining Long-Term Residential Care: An International Study of Promising Practices. Most of her research relies primarily on the perspectives of those who actually provide or manage care within the health care system. In addition to her academic pursuits, Pat Armstrong is involved in a number of civil society organizations and is a board member of both the Canadian Health Coalition and the Canadian Centre for Policy Alternatives.*

National Experts
Pat Armstrong

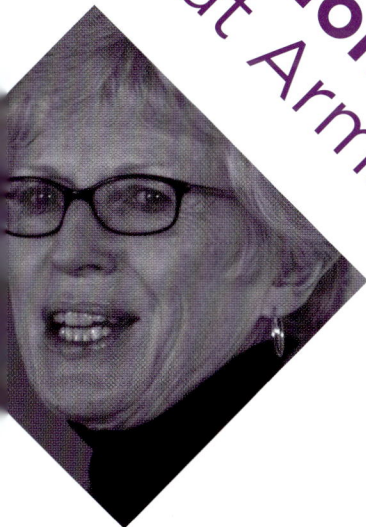

Chapter 3

What do you see as the key issues in continuing care or long-term care?

We have just received funding for a huge project titled, Re-imagining Long-Term Residential Care, and the four big areas we identified are: models of care, work organization, accountability, and financing and ownership. It seems to me those are critical areas for thinking about care.

Why do you think there's been so little debate about long-term care among policy makers and the public?

The history of long-term care is of it being a place for the poor and indigent, the place of last resort, and where we send people to die. So this structures the way we think, and our main idea has been how to keep people out of these facilities, rather than to see them as an integral part of a continuum of care. I can't tell you the number of times people have said to me, "we had to put our mother in a home." With neo-liberal ideology, the dominant thinking is that we are responsible for ourselves and for our families, so if a relative ends up in a facility, everybody feels guilty and awful. We have the idea that the "good" person looks after him or herself, or the family does, especially around personal care — toilet, washing, brushing teeth, combing hair. So this idea about failure, I think, leaks into all the ways we approach these facilities.

Long-term care was never part of the Canada Health Act. *Can you tell me about that?*

After medicare was introduced, people who required a lot of daily care were in hospitals, but we also had chronic care, rehabilitation and psychiatric hospitals that housed an awful lot of other people. With the dramatic reduction in these types of hospitals — all in the name of saving money and because of a belief that institutions are bad — we have ended up with facilities now being the last resort. And to save money and shift costs, the hospitals — which the *Canada Health Act* says have to be free of charge — now send people home quicker and sicker. The [1964] Royal Commission on Health Services said that the only way you will get efficient allocation in care, that is appropriate for the people and economically efficient, is by including [in medicare] the entire range of services, and we haven't done that from the beginning.

Where do you stand on the issue of home care?

I would argue that we need to think of a range of services, that people have options, and we should not think that care in the home is cheaper — it isn't necessarily, and to the extent that it is, it's because we rely on unpaid caregivers: we conscript women into providing care. And I am not convinced it is always the best place. It can be bloody lonely and isolating, it can be scary to be all by oneself, and it can be dangerous. We pretend that there is no granny bashing going on, but there is, so let us not say aging in place is this great panacea. It is more efficient to group people together to provide services rather than have home care workers paid to travel 30 kilometres or half an hour between home care visits and to leave people alone at night. It doesn't have to be in horrible facilities and you could provide better working conditions for those providing care if they didn't have to tramp all over the country and not be paid in between. On the other hand, I think there is another sense in which aging in place is important. To retain peoples' social connections and their identities, the facilities need to be located close to where they live. And if we are really serious about wanting people to age in place, we've got to keep communities intact — for example access to banks, and pharmacies. I think of my 93-year-old father in Northern Ontario. He lives there alone, and he couldn't live there if he couldn't purchase his basic needs within walking distance.

You say it is more cost-effective to group people together in a more humane way than we are now, but I think some would speak differently about aging in place. Is there a tension there?

Sure, and I wouldn't say put everybody in an institution — that is why we use the word *facility* rather than *institution*. But I would argue that we need to think of a range of services to ensure people have options, and we should not think that care at home is cheaper, because it isn't necessarily. When we think of aging in place and home care, we think of a middle-class home where you have easy access to what you need.

What does the evidence say about continuing care and long-term care?

The evidence says that care should not be provided by for-profit companies. The evidence also says the conditions of work are the conditions for care, and we have to pay attention to what happens to the people who work in care. The evidence says you can do things differently: for example, the level of violence in long-term care reported in Nordic countries is seven times less than in Canada, suggesting that you can create different conditions for care. I would argue that the violence here reflects the inadequacy of care — that there is so much difference suggests that this is not about the nature of patients, but rather about how we organize the care. The evidence suggests that reorganizing the services to provide a better kind of continuum of care isn't necessarily a hugely increased expense. And the other thing evidence shows is that this is skilled work. The recognition of the skill that is required shouldn't be ignored.

Can you tell us more about differences between here and the Nordic countries?

I was in Sweden and asked our host to show us a long-term care facility. We walked through a neighbourhood in Stockholm, made up mostly of three- or four-storey apartments and condos, and she said, "Let me see if I can find one." We went through the lobbies of 10 buildings, looking, and she finally identified one only by going into the lobby and reading the signage. Here you can recognize a facility from miles away — they look like mini hospitals and usually have a horrible name. The difference between here and there suggests a very different philosophy. They have really moved towards trying to ensure everyone has their own apartment, even those with severe health issues. For those with dementia, the stove is turned off so they can't harm themselves. There are small common spaces for dining, instead of huge dining halls.

What would you like to see on the agenda if there were a public forum on this issue?

The whole question of how we think about long-term care should be on the agenda. It is very hard to get into these conversations without stepping back and asking what do we mean? What do we think is included, who should be providing care, how should it be provided, whose responsibility is it? What is the individual responsible for, what is the family responsible for? What are the needs of strangers? And I think we need to talk about work organization, which includes all the questions about skill mix, about who is appropriate to provide care — and this has to include unpaid care. It is incredible to me that we teach someone to be a nurse in four years of university and expect them to take five minutes to teach some unpaid caregiver to clean a catheter — something they themselves have taken a week to learn.

Any final thoughts?

We have to dare to dream and not start with the position that we can't do *something*.

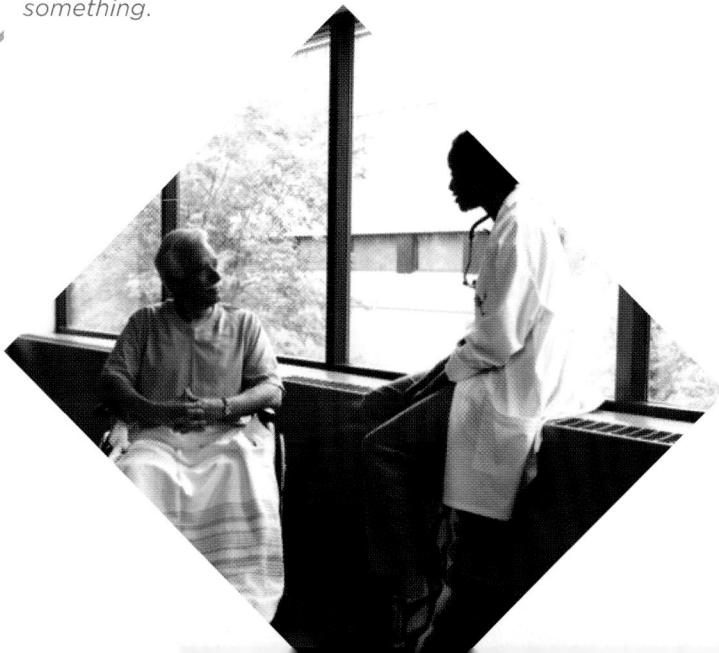

Out of Control: Violence Against Personal Support Workers in Long-Term Care

Led by York University researchers including Pat Armstrong, the study report found:

"The level of violence in Canadian long-term care facilities is extraordinary. Canadian personal support workers are almost seven times more likely to experience violence on a daily basis than workers in Nordic countries. Working short-staffed, a major contributor to the issue is common in Canada but less so in Nordic countries. Nordic long-term care workers also experience greater flexibility on the job and greater communication among colleagues."

The recommendations include:

- Governments must recognize chronic short-staffing is a key contributor to workplace violence and address it by legislating and funding adequate care standards.
- Training must be accessible, designed with worker input, credentialized, and comprehensive.
- Long-term care must be recognized as an essential health service and become a national priority.

Banerjee, A., Daly, T., Armstrong, H., Armstrong, P., Lafrance, S. & Szebehely, M. (2008). *Out of Control: Violence Against Personal Support Workers in Long-Term Care.* Retrieved from: http://www.yorku.ca/mediar/special/out_of_control___english.pdf

Wendy Armstrong

Wendy Armstrong is an independent researcher, policy analyst and consultant based in Edmonton, Alberta. She has written extensively on the privately financed side of health care in Canada and has a particular interest in the evaluation and marketing of new health care-related technologies. As president and executive director of the Consumers' Association of Canada (Alberta Chapter) for much of the 1990s, Armstrong is most well known for her influential 2000 report, The Consumer Experience with Cataract Surgery and Private Clinics in Alberta: Canada's Canary in the Mine Shaft *(www.albertaconsumers.org). During the past decade, her published research has focused on the chronic care landscape and the introduction of assisted living facilities in Alberta. She is currently a member of the board of PharmaWatch and the Alberta Consumers' Association. Armstrong refers to today's hospitals as "drive-through surgery centres with attached emergency departments" because of the cutbacks in beds and services.*

National Experts
Wendy Armstrong

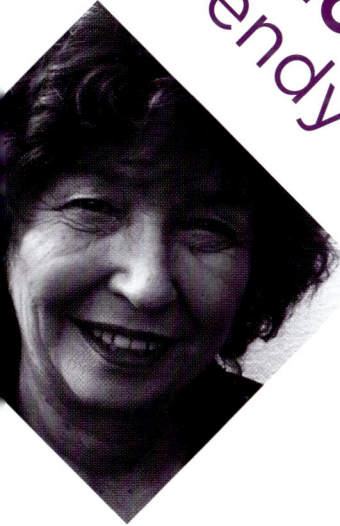

Chapter   4

What do you see as the key issues in continuing care for seniors today?

Seniors have been hit by a double whammy. There is less support for their ongoing care needs and far less for their acute care needs. In the late 80s, there was a groundswell of support for seniors wanting more patient-friendly options — less institutional care, more home-like settings. The plan was a dramatic ramp up of home care and community programs, such as day programs for the elderly, and more social housing models. And we started some interesting and good models. But early on, it became apparent how the models shifted responsibilities and costs onto unprepared families. Everybody has this fantasy that all seniors who require care live in paid-off houses with lots of assets, but in reality these extra charges can create a disincentive for individuals to go into programs. And then in 1991, they started downsizing the hospitals and increasing the number of day surgeries. If you were admitted, you were discharged quicker and sicker. This is a huge national issue. Home care suddenly became the domain of short-term recovery — resources went to caring for people discharged after very short hospital stays.

I understand Alberta began promoting assisted living in a big way and that this approach is also spreading to other provinces. Can you explain what it is?

This is the new substitute model for traditional long-term care. It is *à la carte* care. People think of it as a location but it is actually a program [and] it is the false promise of aging in place. The idea is that you go in when you are well and then care can be added on as needed. You have to be willing and able to pay additional costs. But the most important thing, that is so hard to wrap your mind around, is that it is about the unbundling of care. There are a lot more co-payments or outright expenses. For example, residents can face out-of-pocket charges for medication assistance, night checks, meal escorts, assistance with support stockings, incontinence management and bath assistance. When I did the research and understood what was coming, I desperately tried to explain this paradigm shift, and people said, 'What do you mean, they will charge me extra to respond to an emergency call bell?' It is like they waved pixie dust and zap, nursing care became residential care. So now administering meds goes from health care professionals to the housing operator — and one new cost for residents is that now they have to pay extra to have their pills in blister packs [for ease of administration by nonprofessionals]. Meanwhile, the letters that families get from politicians imply that this model empowers residents to have a choice, and if they don't like it they can move, but [it is ridiculous] to suggest that bedridden people being tube-fed have this option.

But long-term care was never covered in medicare and is not part of the Canada Health Act.

True, but the difference now is this new kind of emphasis on the individual paying. Our medicare system was not set up so that the public health plan pays for everything you need. But we did have this concept that once you reached a certain level of need, we should all share in the costs of that need. This concept is being quietly dismantled. For example, high-needs individuals used to be in chronic care hospitals. We had expected a housing model where care needs would be fully funded by the public, but this was hijacked by other agendas, and here in Alberta it was to make room for the private sector and private real estate development. Seniors housing has more to do with real estate than with care; everyone wants to get in on the seniors' boom market. And now there is a real shortage of affordable care for high-needs people, while there is a glut of high-end assisted living facilities. There is an absolute disconnect.

What do you think we need to better understand?

What we need to understand is that the issue of continuing care cannot be looked at in isolation from what is happening with housing, income security and early discharges from acute care. We need to see the whole context. And this is fundamentally not just about senior citizens who need care, but also about the sustainability of families — emotionally and financially. We need to understand that this is a family issue. The reality is that the children of seniors may live hundreds of miles away and not be able to themselves provide the extra care that is needed on a temporary or more permanent basis; some adult children are taking second jobs so they can pay for the services needed by their aging parents. Meanwhile, we are putting so much time and money into assessment tools and data collection that RNs have little time left for direct care. Marshall McLuhan [the Canadian theorist] said that our tools shape us: I am struck by the fact that when more money is available, so much of it is diverted to information management and so much time and effort goes into collecting statistics — at the expense of direct care. It's not that we don't need data collection, but what is happening is like data collection on steroids.

What is your prescription for the future?

I can't think of anything more important for 40-year-olds to unite on than to ensure adequate care for their parents, for the short or long term. We need care as much in Vancouver as in St. John's. We need to understand that if we don't pay collectively through our taxes, all that means is that you will have to quit your job, or work part time, or impoverish yourself to care for your parents. Until recently, in some provinces, spouses had to sell their assets and live in poverty if they had a partner in care. Unfortunately, language makes it almost impossible to have national debates: we don't know what each other is talking about. It took me a long time to figure out how British Columbia was different from Alberta — we had *public lodges, nursing homes* and *auxiliary hospitals* while they had *nursing homes* with *multiple layers of care.* And every time a new report comes out, there is new language.

For Patients' Sake: Patient First Review

"Patients ask that health care workers and their respective leadership see beyond their declared interests so that the interest of patients takes precedence at every care interaction, every future contract negotiation and every policy debate."

The report found that "seniors needing long-term care are ill-served by a system that leaves them in hospital beds, without the requisite supports and programming, while awaiting placement in an appropriate facility. The financial, physical and emotional costs can be significant, and at times overwhelming, for the individual, their spouse and family."

The commissioner recommended that the Ministry of Health's Seniors' Strategy under development focuses on strengthening:

a) System capacity to support independent living;
b) Accessibility to personal care homes by addressing the current financial barriers for low-income seniors;
c) Accessibility and quality of assisted living and long-term care;
d) Programming for seniors with extraordinary behaviours that cannot be safely managed in the general long-term care; and
e) Capacity of geriatric assessment programs to provide multidisciplinary assessments, short-term rehabilitation, day programs, and a specialized outpatient clinic.

Dagnone, T. (October, 2009). *For Patients' Sake: Patient First Review Commissioner's Report to the Saskatchewan Minister of Health.* Retrieved from: http://www.health.gov.sk.ca/patient-first-commissioners-report

Dr. Margaret McGregor

Dr. Margaret McGregor is a family physician at the Mid-Main Community Health Centre in Vancouver and a researcher with a special interest in how nursing homes vary depending on who owns them and how they are organized. Her research is supported in part through a Vancouver Foundation grant to the Department of Family Practice at the University of British Columbia, where she is clinical associate professor. The grant enables her, as a community-based clinician investigator, to spend time with her patients and also conduct research. Dr. McGregor is a co-investigator in an ongoing research project that aims to improve communication and collaboration between home health staff and general practitioners, with the goal of improving care for patient/clients. In addition to her other roles, Dr. McGregor is a research associate at the Vancouver Coastal Health Research Institute's Centre for Clinical Epidemiology and Evaluation and UBC's Centre for Health Services and Policy Research.

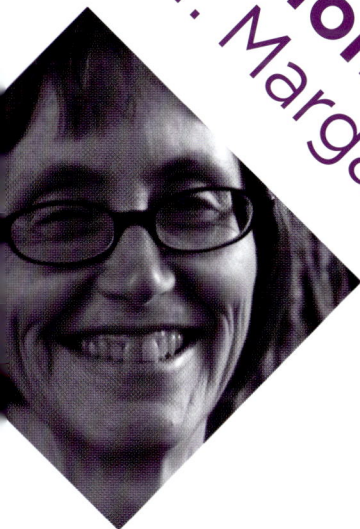

National Experts
Dr. Margaret McGregor

I know much of your research has been into long-term care facilities. What do you think are the key issues we are facing in Canada?

I do think the broad issue is how we can best address the needs of the aging population. Clearly, even if people age with better function than they did in the past, there will be a need for more residential long-term care and other forms of senior housing. So then the question is, how is that expansion of capacity going to take place? Based on the literature reviewed and my own research, there is sufficient empirical evidence to conclude that public funding to private for-profit facilities is likely to produce inferior quality. This does not mean that all for-profit facilities provide inferior care, nor that all non-profit and public facilities provide superior care. However, the evidence tells us that, as a group, private for-profit facilities are likely to have inferior quality compared to public or non-profit facilities. It is therefore wise for public policy to reflect this evidence. Unfortunately, the policy direction in many provinces has been to build new facilities using P3s, or public-private partnerships. This results in care being delivered in the for-profit sector, which is not consistent with the evidence.

Tell me more about P3s. I understand British Columbia has gone into that in a big way.

P3s are agreements between the contractor, in this case the government, and a private company. In the case of residential care, the care is then publicly funded but delivered by the private for-profit company that constructed the facility or by one of its affiliates.

The P3s and methods of funding do seem to anchor the for-profits for quite a while. I expect they are hard deals to get out of.

Yes, as the CUPE report [*Residential Long-Term Care in Canada: Our Vision for Better Seniors' Care*, 2009] points out, these contracts are often for very long terms and difficult to get out of.

How can government increase accountability of facilities to provide good care?

One way to do this is by having good regulations in place. Another strategy is to provide the public with facility data on complaints and inspection reports as Ontario has done. But such systems are expensive. For example, in the US, which is highly regulated, the annual cost of running state licensing agencies is estimated to be $22,000 per facility, or $208 per bed.

Are there alternative ways of financing new construction?

Governments can sell bonds to raise capital for residential care — this is done quite a bit in the United States, and Alberta is getting into it. The Canadian Healthcare Association is calling for a non-profit social insurance scheme that younger people could buy into, something that is quite common in Europe.

I notice that your research reveals differences among the non-profit facilities — those that are connected to a hospital or health authority, or that have more than one site of operation, send fewer residents to hospital for conditions such as pneumonia and dehydration.

That is correct. In BC we found that overall the non-profit sector fares better than the for-profit, but there clearly are also differences between the not-for-profits in larger groupings and the others. The reasons for those differences merit more research. There is not a lot of good Canadian research yet on differences among non-profits, even though apart from Ontario, the majority of service delivery in Canada remains in that sector.

Why isn't there more research?

Generally speaking, research into residential long-term care doesn't get funded at the same level as drug trials and new technologies. Researchers need to develop an interest in this area, and policymakers and funders need to encourage research. But while more research is needed to explore differences within the non-profit sector, I don't think this should stop governments from generally supporting policies that nurture non-profit and public delivery — there is already enough evidence on that question.

What other factors have you observed that make a difference to the quality of continuing care?

Based on my clinical experience, the integration of primary medical care — family doctors — into residential care is an important issue. Often they are worlds apart. Facilities where there is a system of house physicians who regularly attend care conferences seem to do better, have lower rates of transfer to hospital and are able to provide better end-of-life care and support for families. Good delivery of end-of-life care is an important discussion that needs to be encouraged. This is a population that is frail. The average length of stay of residents at an extended care level facility is now about 18 months in some provinces. So it's important to figure out ways to help facilities provide good comfort care at the end of life. We recently completed a study where we found that the only factor that seemed to be associated with a facility's decision not to transfer a resident from extended care to hospital near the end of life was having the continuity of a regular family doctor who cared for residents from the time of admission to death. That continuity of care seemed to matter in some way, presumably because trusting relationships develop over time and allow for important conversations about end-of-life care. So integrating primary medical care into the team would be quite important to improving how we do residential long-term care.

What are your prescriptions for the future?

I would like to see Canada really ramp up public sources of funding for facility construction either through traditional public sector funding, bond sales, or financing from public agencies such as the Canada Mortgage and Housing Corporation. On the delivery side, I'd like to see governments develop infrastructure to support not-for-profit groups to be able to respond to RFPs [requests for proposals] to construct facilities that are competitive. These RFPs should also develop scoring systems that take into account the social capital that non-profit groups provide. A lot of requests for proposals are all about efficiency and providing service for lower cost; they don't measure the things that are harder to measure, like the extent to which a not-for-profit society has good community roots, and whether they are able to mobilize volunteers. A scoring system should recognize those properties, and not simply who delivers the lowest-cost care.

Anything else?

I think it is important to develop a team approach to care. There is evidence that when leadership listens to and respects team work, quality is better. Health care aides, for instance, often get left out of care conferences, yet they play such an important role — as front-line staff they are often the eyes and ears of residents, and have a much better sense of where residents are at by virtue of spending more time with them. Another important policy direction would be to improve the alignment of the acute care and residential long-term care sectors so that hospitals "adopt" the residential care facilities in their catchment area and there is a much stronger sense of mutual accountability. It should be standard practice for anyone transferring a resident to an emergency room to have a conversation with the emergency room doctor who is accepting the resident. In the same way, a patient should not be discharged from hospital back to a continuing care facility without a conversation with the facility about the patient's treatment and experiences in hospital.

Community Indicators for an Aging Population

Overarching findings from research indicate that:

"Most Canadian communities have made minimal progress in achieving smart growth and livability goals to date, and are thus ill-prepared to accommodate the housing and mobility needs of an aging population. Government leadership is needed to… push these issues to the forefront of the public policy agenda."

Canadian Mortgage and Housing Corporation. (2008). *Research Highlight: Community Indicators for an Aging Population.* Retrieved from: http://www.cmhc-schl.gc.ca/odpub/pdf/66099.pdf

Josephine Etowa

Josephine Etowa is a co-author of Anti-Racist Health Care Practice *(Canadian Scholars' Press Inc., 2009) and has more than twenty-three years of clinical practice in the areas of maternal and newborn health, and inequity in health and health care. An associate professor at the University of Ottawa's School of Nursing, she has conducted extensive research in the area of women's health and diversity in the health care system. Her research projects have been funded by international, national and provincial agencies and are based on the principles of qualitative research and participatory action research. Etowa is a founding member of the Health Association of African Canadians and has been involved in a number of community development initiatives to improve knowledge about African Canadians' health. She began her career as a midwife and public health nurse in Nigeria.*

National Experts
Josephine Etowa

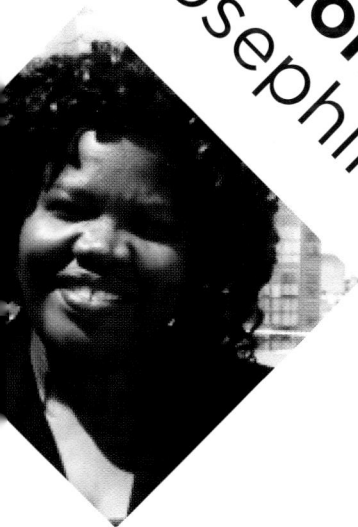

Chapter 6

One of your areas of research is diversity in the workplace. How did you get interested?

When I first moved to Canada, like many immigrants I worked in home care and also in a long-term care facility. I was already trained as a nurse and midwife, but I was employed as a personal care worker while I was preparing for my RN exams. Some of my patients had never had to interact with Black people, and the most challenging work was home care because patients would do things they wouldn't do in public. Some people said "don't touch me," or they complained, saying I could not speak English. Some patients hit me really hard. One woman chased me out of her house in her wheelchair; I just ran out crying. When she complained, the office told her I was overqualified. I went back to her, and eventually we became friends, and she always asked for me to be her caregiver. But it took me proving that beyond the Black skin was a very good nurse.

How did you deal with this?

On one hand, you understand what they feel — they had never had to deal with someone they considered inferior, and they were being forced to have very intimate contact. It's a complex issue. Maybe we cannot change the older population today, but we can change the new ones coming along by starting integration early, so that in nursing training — and in law, in medicine — we have people interacting from diverse backgrounds so that by the time they get to the workforce it is not an issue. When I started out here in Canada, there was no adequate training about cultural competence.

Have you seen much progress?

The issue is getting some attention, but even now there is not much cultural competence training for health care providers who have to work across ethno-cultural boundaries. The Canadian demographic is changing and we need to keep up with this. We need diversity in training programs so all long-term care nurses go through some cultural competence training, and there should be something like accreditation that mandates institutions to show evidence of what they are doing around this issue. From my own study of the worklife of visible minority nurses — including Black, Asian, Indian, Hispanic, and my most recent study looking at Aboriginal nurses — there is consistent talk about the lack of cultural competence, about patients being treated inadequately and inappropriately. And when you see patients treated like that, you think: that could be your mom or dad.

The relative of a friend of mine, a gay man, was dying, and my friend told me he was so relieved to finally have a gay male nurse. He had been uncomfortable with previous nurses.

What I find in my research, it is not so much that patients need someone who looks like them, but someone who is competent and who understands their culture. But in the absence of that, you do want someone like you because it is easier to start a dialogue. The issue is how we can train health care providers to be open to diversity — to gay people, to poor people, to people with different skin colours. And sometimes it is also about images in institutions: in long-term care, do you see images that speak to you? Do you feel welcome?

What are some of the practical issues that come up?

When you come in as a visible minority patient, quite often your needs are not met. For example, nurses have not been taught how to find a vein in dark-skinned people, or how to assess for anaemia. And I try to see things as teaching moments. Some of my students said they found my accent difficult. I said fine, let's set ground rules: we need to decode other peoples' accents, so the university is giving you an advantage here: you will learn to decode. Even my colleagues, the first time I had braids in my hair, I used that as a teaching moment so at least when they saw the next patient with braids, they wouldn't think the person was not well cared for. So if you have a level of interaction, it exposes you to that culture.

What kind of initiatives have you seen around cultural competence?

In May this year [2010], there was a national trans-cultural health conference in Calgary and we actually had a dialogue about national standards on cultural competence. I was in Nova Scotia until a year ago and I served on a number of committees on primary health care renewal. Nova Scotia had the first cultural competence guidelines in 2007 around primary health. At Dalhousie University, once we got diversity into the mission statement, and then the strategic direction, it had to be addressed. We created a committee and a program for recruitment and retention and we increased the enrolment of Black nursing students by 200%. When something is in a mission statement and a committee is created, people put targeted effort towards it.

What about research into diversity in long-term care?

Of course we need more research. We don't have enough research in other areas, like medicine, and even less in home care or long-term care. Of course long-term care is already marginalized, so it suffers double jeopardy.

Diversity Our Strength: LGBT Tool Kit For Creating Lesbian, Gay, Bisexual and Transgendered Culturally Competent Care at Toronto Long-Term Care Homes and Services

"Many LGBT seniors report heightened fear and anxiety should they disclose their sexual orientation to service providers within both health and social service agencies and have little faith and confidence that they would not experience further victimization. Within current literature and research, it is indicated that LGBT elders are five times less likely to use services than the population at large as a result of this fear."

In Toronto, a Tool Kit was developed to help guide and establish cultural competencies in providing long-term care and services for LGBT residents, their partners, and their friends, while also creating a welcoming environment for volunteers, staff and the local community who comes in contact with the homes and programs.

"Cultural competence is defined as a set of congruent behaviors, attitudes, and policies that come together in a system, agency, or among professionals and enables the system, agency, or those professionals to work effectively in cross-cultural situations."

The Tool Kit focuses on six areas: Welcoming Environment; Nursing and Personal Care; Administrative Processes; Staff and Volunteers; Programs and Services; and Community Engagement.

Toronto Long-Term Care Homes & Services. (2008). *Diversity Our Strength: LGBT Tool Kit For Creating Lesbian, Gay, Bisexual and Transgendered Culturally Competent Care at Toronto Long-Term Care Homes and Services.* Toronto: Author. Retrieved from: http://www.toronto.ca/ltc/lgbt_toolkit.htm

Sheila Neysmith

Sheila Neysmith, a professor in the Faculty of Social Work at the University of Toronto, has published extensively on how public policies affect the caring labour that women do throughout their lives. She is currently the principal investigator on an international comparative study of promising practices in home care. Her books include Critical Issues for Future Social Work Practice with Aging Persons *(1999), and she is a co-author of* Beyond Caring Labour to Provisioning Work *(University of Toronto Press, forthcoming). For several years, Neysmith directed the Graduate Collaborative Program in Women's Studies for the University of Toronto. During that time she co-edited* Feminist Utopias: Re-Visioning our Futures *(2002). She has been a member of the management team for the China Project for a number of years, editing with Liu Meng and Xiaobei Chen* Women and Social Work in China *(2007).*

National Experts
Sheila Neysmith

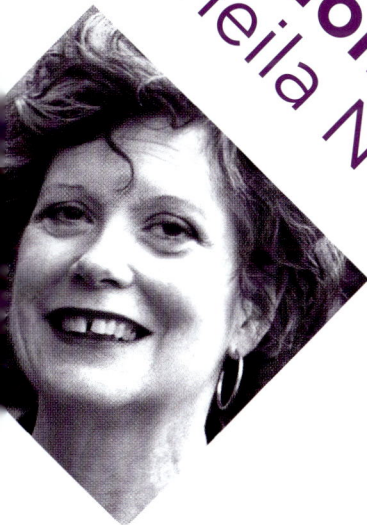

Chapter 7

What do you see as the key issues in continuing care in Canada?

I think the emphasis needs to be on the time before people need long-term care. We need to go upstream, so not as many people need to go into long-term care. From my standpoint, there's abundant evidence now that home care is cost-effective and desired by people for a number of stages of disability until they are in such bad shape that, by anyone's standards including their own, they have to go into a nursing home. But before that, you need various levels of home care. So my question is, since we are always talking about evidence-based policy, how come the home care policy has never moved in Canada? For comparison, in Australia they have had a national home and community care policy since 1986.

Why do you think we don't have a more developed home care strategy?

We devote very little energy, let alone money, to supportive home care — the type of care that people can routinely expect as they get older, that will increase their quality of life. Some will argue home care dollars have increased, and that is true, but money is being used to attend to hospital budget problems. In the mid-90s, to deal with hospital budget problems, they started having people leave hospital earlier, and what limited home care budget there was got used for post-acute patients at home. This trend to accommodate hospitals is particularly strong in Ontario where the Aging at Home Strategy is moving into its third year. Its key evaluating criteria includes the degree to which it addresses the issue of people waiting in hospital to get into long-term care, and the use of emergency department services for older people. Meanwhile, even as home care service dollars have increased, services that involve personal support workers who come in and help the frail elderly with activities of daily living have been cut. This is an issue across the country. I know chapter and verse in terms of Ontario, but this taking over of the home care agenda by the medical agenda is an issue across the country.

What is the impact of this focus on the needs of the acute care sector?

There's all this talk about the post-World War II cohort [baby boomers] coming through and how expensive this is going to be. But it is not that these aging people are causing the expense, it is how we organize the services. It is the technology and organization of health care that leads to rising health care costs, not the aging of the population. We continue to use dollars in health care for purchasing medical-like services, and so the hospital sector will indeed continue to develop unless we put in place a policy that actually steers money into the development of home care services.

How did Australia manage to develop and protect supportive home care services?

I think they recognized that if you put money into a health care budget and you have a powerful hospital sector, the big guys [in the hospital sector] will always win the game. So they red-circled a certain percentage of the heath care budget, about two percent to three percent, and told the states that if they want to develop home and community care services, the Commonwealth would match the money with the red-circled money. But if they didn't use it for home and community care, it couldn't be used for hospitals and it would go back to general revenues. I am not saying this is feasible in the current political atmosphere in Canada, but my basic argument is that if there is a will to try to figure out federal/provincial relations, there is a way.

Some people will argue that staying at home as you age is not really so great.

Home is not always a great place, absolutely it is not. But many people have attachments to their homes. It may not be the best place for them, but they have the right to live in at-risk circumstances if they choose to live at home and could go somewhere else — if, hypothetically, some kind of affordable supportive living situation was available. Home care is still a relatively efficient and cost-effective way to deliver care. So I say, if you chose to live at home, the least I can provide is a couple of hours a day of home help to make sure you get some food and get to the bathroom and that sort of stuff. Currently, I am a kind of follow-along researcher to House Calls, a pilot project where a team of people goes into the homes of really frail elderly people, and I would say of the close to 200 clients, there would probably be about five who would say their choice would be to go into supportive housing.

I think you have said that the lack of supportive home care fosters the growth of for-profit alternatives — correct?

This is a huge, a huge issue. We have this two-class system. If you have the resources, you can buy into the private market, either by hiring the equivalent of personal care workers by the hour — there is a huge market of private agencies that hire out personal service workers by the hour — or moving to a retirement home. But in neither option is there any real quality control. If you live outside the city, there is not much choice and it is *buyer beware.* And not everyone can afford to pay for care. God forbid you are somewhere in the large middle between being independent and needing high levels of care.

What are your prescriptions for the future?

I don't think the answers are all going to be in a unidirectional push. I am also moving along the age dimension, and people talk about getting together and organizing a small edition of the (Toronto) Older Women's Network, with their co-op housing approach, but not everybody is into that kind of organizing mode. I would like to see something like House Calls — a multidisciplinary team that works within a geographic area and supports frail older people who live at home. And we need to acknowledge the huge diversity in our population. I work closely with a Chinese group called Carefirst, and their home care workers are all fluent in Mandarin or

Cantonese so the elders can talk to them. I think we have to recognize that with home care, it is the relationship part — not just the tasks — that allows the work to be done.

You sound a bit hopeful and quite a bit frustrated.

The debate around supportive home care is absolutely silent and off the stage — purposely kept off the stage while the big players play in terms of money. Nobody is talking about a serious move to get supportive home care up and going; always something else takes priority. There needs to be an upping of the volume of a policy debate. Change does not happen from the top, there are points of privilege and power in there that profit again from the status quo. If the needed changes are going to come, they will have to be from various advocacy groups that push on this.

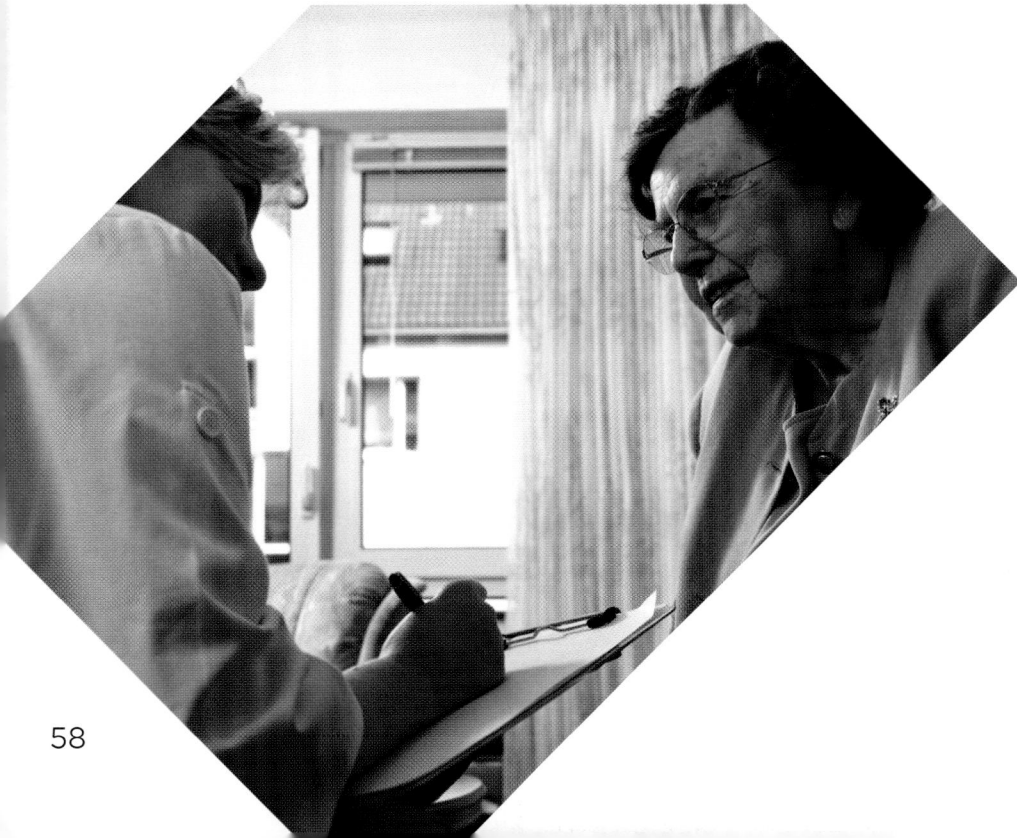

The Long-Term Care Environment: Improving Outcomes Through Staffing Decisions

The Canadian Nurses Association believes that health care reform must include broad policy around housing, healthy aging and income support. In 2008, they published a policy brief specific to long-term care.

- 560,000 to 740,000 seniors will need placement in a long-term care (LTC) facility by 2031.

- There is a wide range of approaches to funding, delivering and regulating LTC throughout the country.

- Inadequate staffing levels in LTC facilities contribute to high rates of violence against health care providers as well as issues around quality of patient care.

- The addition of nurse practitioners in LTC facilities has averted the need to transfer patients to acute care.

- Increased access to on-the-job training and education helps improve work environments and supports safe and quality care.

Canadian Nurses Association. (2008). *The Long-Term Care Environment: Improving Outcomes Through Staffing Decisions.* Ottawa: Author. Retrieved from: http://www.cna-aiic.ca/CNA/documents/pdf/publications/HHR_Policy_Brief4_2008_e.pdf

Today BC's seniors have less access to care and are asked to pay more for the care they receive. Since 2001, the population of seniors over 85 in BC has increased by 43%, yet by 2008, we had the second lowest rate of access to care for people over 75 in the country. By 2003, BC had gone from being a leader in providing home health services to spending well below the national average on these services.

Piled on top of the increased need for public services is the current government's stubborn promotion of private care and user pay options. Despite evidence that private, for-profit facilities provide a lower standard of care, since 2001, private for-profit residential care facilities have grown by 20% in BC and public not-for-profits have declined by 11%. New and increased fees on the sick, recovering and elderly in care are introduced regularly. BC's families deserve much better.

Debra McPherson
President, British Columbia Nurses' Union (BCNU)

Provincial View
Marcia Carr

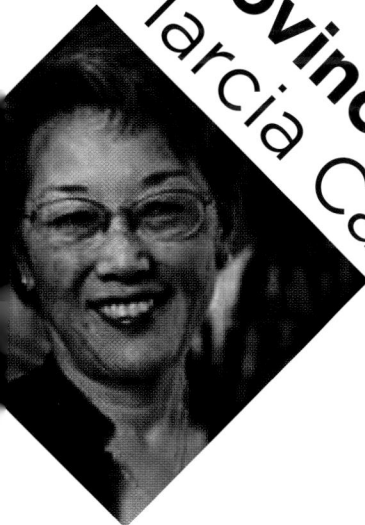

Chapter 8

Charges for necessary health care leave older Canadians vulnerable and may well amount to a "system-level type of elder abuse or neglect" if patients can't access services and treatments because they are unable to pay, says Marcia Carr, a clinical nurse specialist at the Fraser Health Older Adult Program in British Columbia.

For example, some patients discharged from hospital need additional rehabilitation and recovery time in order to regain a safe level of functioning and mobility. But health authorities in British Columbia are implementing various new charges for services that adversely impact on older adults — they are given the choice of paying for their rehabilitation or convalescent care stay in a health authority designated facility, or returning home with or without services, she says. Although there is a sliding scale charge based on income for either facility or at-home services, individuals often decide to return home without receiving convalescent care because the cost imposes a financial burden on them. "Services are supposed to be there when you are ill and you need help — right care, right provider, right place and in a timely manner," Carr notes.

"If that older adult is already paying for their own apartment, how are they going to find the money to pay for their recovery?" Seniors can apply for hardship funding, but there's no guarantee that they will receive it. "Is it respectful care to ask older adults to be assessed for hardship?"

Patients who return home directly, instead of going to convalescent care, might be able to receive some rehabilitation. "But it wouldn't be the same intensity, to say the least. And for every day an older adult is in bed, they can lose up to 5% of muscle strength," says Carr, who is an adjunct professor in gerontology research at Simon Fraser University and the schools of nursing at the University of British Columbia and the University of Victoria, and a clinical assistant professor at the McMaster University School of Nursing.

Too many elderly Canadians end up in residential care because housekeeping services are no longer provided as part of home health services. "Now they have to privately hire a housekeeping service or have family members, if they are around, do these chores. Many older adults who just need help with housekeeping in order to remain at home may end up harming themselves trying to clean and cook when it is beyond their physical capacity."

Carr is also concerned about the availability of appropriate and timely care. Health authorities in the province are engaging in service re-design and working on strategies to address the increasing care needs of the population. "However, implementation is going forward even though there currently aren't enough beds in care facilities or hospitals, or qualified service providers in the system for the strategies to work now," she says.

For example, when someone fractures a hip, the literature says surgery should take place within a maximum of 48 hours, and preferably within 24 hours — "the longer the wait, the greater the morbidity and mortality." However, wait times for hip surgery in BC can be up to five days or more. "We continue to have delays and long wait times for surgery which result in more complications for patients, such as deep vein thrombosis, delirium, pneumonias, bed sores, and urinary tract infections from Foley catheters." Treating these complications leads to longer hospital stays that, in turn, limit the availability of beds for the next patient who needs the surgery. "There is just this terrible downward cascade that occurs. When a patient develops a delirium, then all the other 'geriatric giants' implode concurrently upon them."

If older adults received time-sensitive surgery and are moved to rehabilitation at the right time, more would be able to return home more quickly. That would free up more hospital beds, enabling more timely surgery to happen. "I don't have data at my fingertips to support that, it just makes common sense," says Carr. Research shows that close to 50% of older adults who fracture a hip and end up in a nursing home will die within a year of admission to the facility. "Why is this outcome acceptable?"

Carr would like to see much more attention paid to preparing all health care providers to care for the population of older Canadians. "Older adults present differently. Health care providers need to be able to differentiate between normal aging and pathology, and they need to know what to do to support functionality. But if you don't know what you don't know, then how are you supposed to even know what to ask? So... guess what? You unknowingly create more problems for the older adults and thus to the system because you have debilitated them prematurely or accelerated their decline while in our care."

For six years, Carr and her clinical nurse specialist colleagues travelled BC with the acute care geriatric nurse network to spread the word about caring for acutely ill older adults and to hear stories from the front lines. For example, after a session about identifying delirium, Carr heard from front-line nurses how critical it is that specific education be provided with respect to properly assessing and caring for patients with delirium and how easily the condition can be misunderstood.

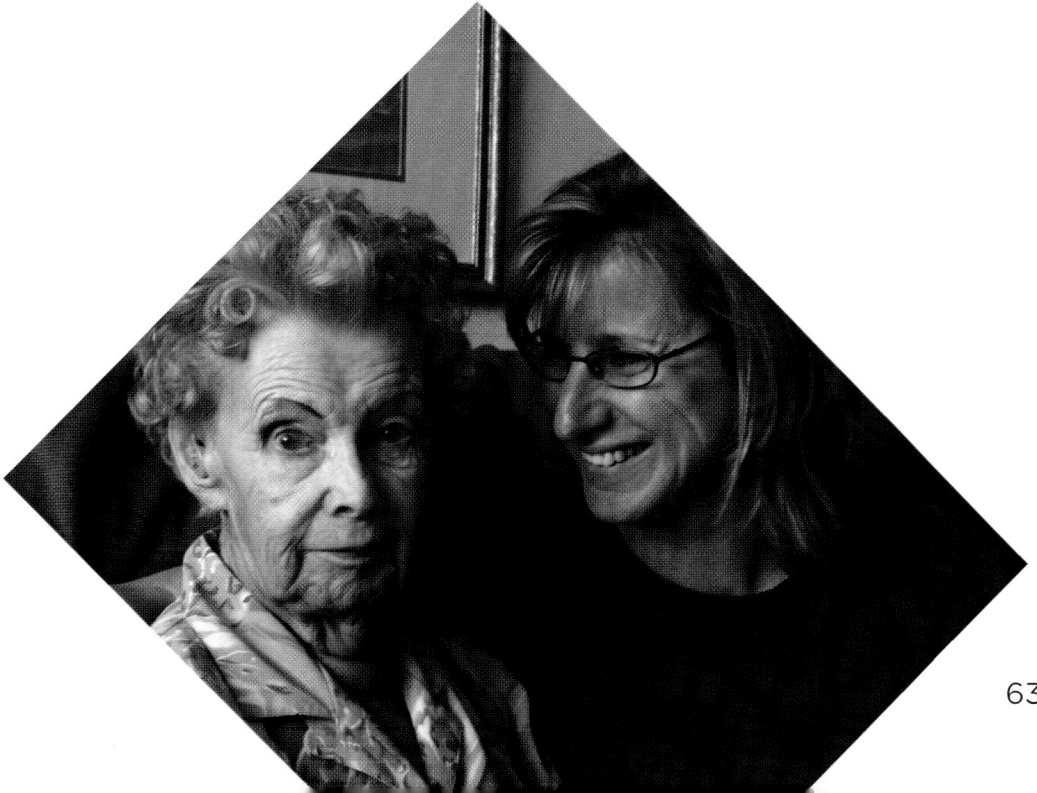

Government keeps changing the language — long-term care is now "continuing care." We have "assisted living" and "designated assisted living." Nursing homes and auxiliary hospitals are redesignated to remove any obligation to provide skilled RNs and LPNs. It's like three-card monte, guess under what shell care is provided — unless you can pay for it.

I have been told of seniors married 50 or 60 years, who are counseled to legally separate because they cannot afford the costs associated with one of the spouses entering a "care" facility. Instead of "assisted living," governments should call them "assisted dying." This is an unconscionable abdication of responsibility and a national shame.

Heather Smith
President, United Nurses of Alberta (UNA)

Provincial View
Karen Kuprys

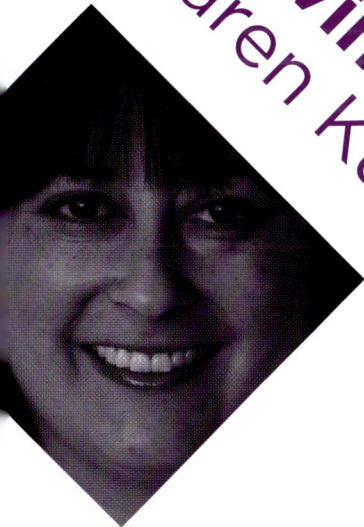

Chapter 9

Baby boomers still have a few years to "turn things around," but only if they open their eyes, see what is happening in care for the elderly — and take political steps to change things. "When they become infirm and elderly, they aren't going to be able to change the system."

That's the warning issued by Karen Kuprys, an Edmonton nurse with certification in gerontology from the Canadian Nurses Association (RN, GNC (C)).

For the past 17 years, Kuprys has worked in institutions with up to 220 residents. "Like at all nursing homes, our acuity has gone up. We have people who are basically medical cases who have been discharged from hospitals."

But instead of beefing up the numbers and qualifications of staff, the opposite is happening. Kuprys now works with two licensed practical nurses on a unit of 50 residents. "I have a med cart and I know everyone," she explains. But already-announced changes will leave her responsible for about 100 residents "doing crisis management" because she will no longer be integrated into the unit.

The problem? The institution where she works, formerly a nursing home, was re-designated as an auxiliary hospital, and staffing requirements disappeared. "If you are designated a nursing home, you need 22% professional component, but in an auxiliary care hospital you can take patients with the same, or higher levels of acuity and not even need any professional staff."

Kuprys observes that although provincial government officials pay lip service to the idea that caring for the elderly is a specialized task, their actions reveal they believe that "anybody can do it."

And she is disheartened at the forthcoming changes: "These are real people that we care for, and they need real, skilled people looking after them, and that includes RNs. It physically hurts me to see what is happening; if these residents were people's children there is no way they would be looked after this way. There would be an outcry about staffing ratios."

Not all residents understand the implications of the changes, but those that do feel powerless, she says. "They are already in the system, and where do you go?"

The key issue for Kuprys is removing the registered nurse from the bedside. "I don't mean every bedside, but being in an office, shuffling paper and directing care, how can a nurse make proper assessments? I mean, nurses don't go into nursing to say 'how can I do the worst job possible?'"

The direction that Alberta is heading in, with the emphasis on assisted living accommodation, is disturbing, she says. At the Alberta Gerontological Nurses Association conference in the spring of 2010, a provincial draft plan was presented that outlined three levels of care at assisted living before people are even eligible for long-term care, she says.

"In assisted living, there will be no registered nurses on site — maybe there will be one on call. RNs would act as case managers for placements. So my question was, if it's true that long-term-care patients are clogging up active treatment beds, if they are assessed as able to go to assisted living, what happens if they get sicker? They either clog up assisted living, or get kicked back to emergency wards — so the plan doesn't solve the problem that there are not enough long-term care beds because the province doesn't want to fund them."

And then there's the issue of additional charges. Kuprys knew an older couple that moved into assisted living accommodation and the overweight woman had a fall. She says that because of the $80 charge for responding to an emergency call bell, the frail husband decided to pick her up himself. "I don't think the public really understands... that assisted living is a way of downloading the costs onto the individual. When you go in, you may not need that much care. But all that needs to happen is for your condition to deteriorate" and then charges go up.

Kuprys suggests that it is not by accident that patients and their families are confused or misled by the terminology that is used to describe various types and levels of care for the elderly. "I think there is a quite purposeful attempt to disrupt the public system, to try to destabilize the system, to convince people the only option is private care."

In a draft discussion paper on the nursing and health care aide (HCA) workforce, circulated in August 2010, Alberta Health Services puts forward, as an option, a significant expansion of "supportive living" arrangements "rather than facility-based long-term care beds," to meet the future demands of Albertans aged 65 years and older. This policy change, the paper stated, would allow for a percentage of registered nurses to be "redeployed to other areas of the continuum of care, thereby more efficiently utilizing RNs reducing the projected shortage slightly." The draft paper also notes that "this requires growth to the HCA workforce in all sectors and changes to the corresponding skill mix ratios."

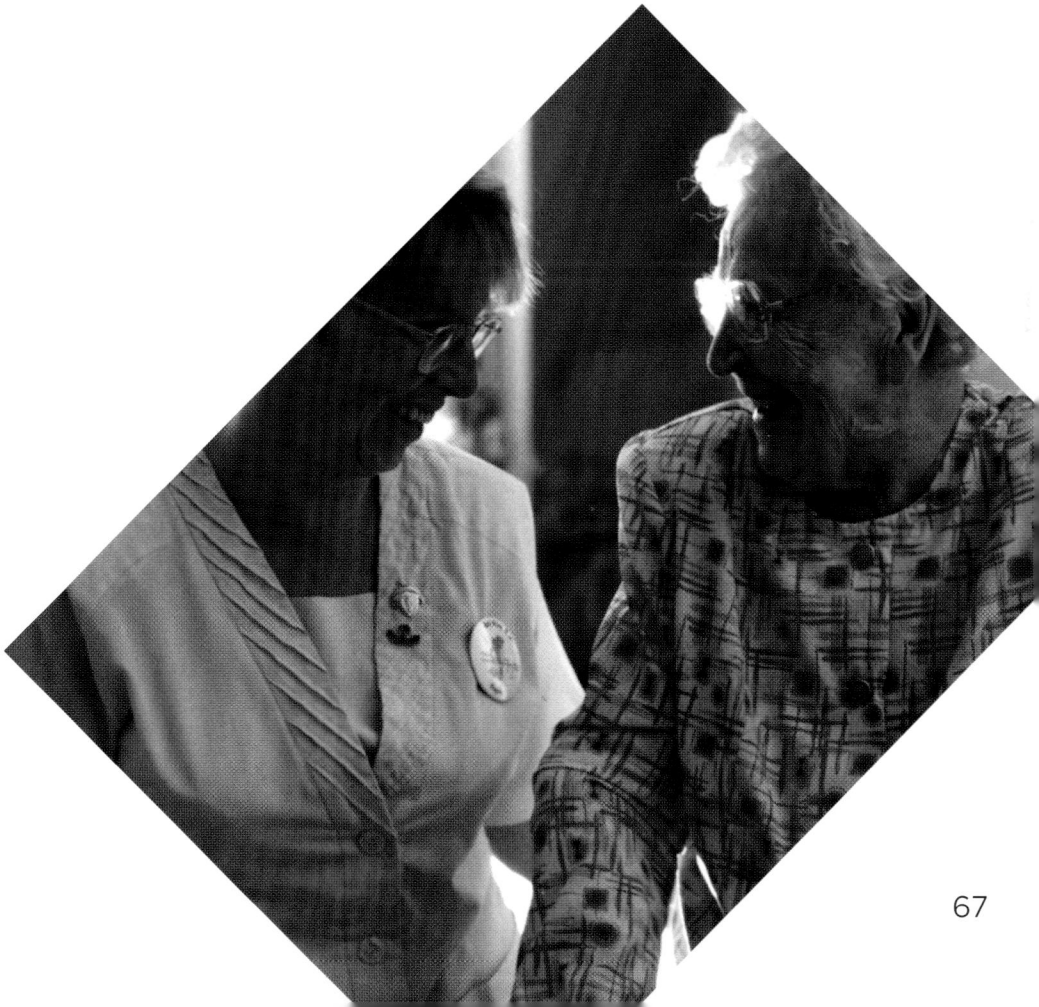

With research and statistics telling us there is going to be a boom in people requiring long-term care, we must focus more attention in this area. Otherwise we will not be ready for their care. Given the increasing complexity and acuity of residents in long-term care, it is going to require a depth and breadth of knowledge and skill that only registered nurses possess. Educating nursing students about this area of health care is going to require a major shift in how universities and colleges deliver their curriculum.

What is urgently needed in long-term care are retention and recruitment strategies with dedicated resources to ensure that registered nurses are being hired and encouraged to stay in the field to lead the team that provides high-quality, patient-centred care.

Rosalee Longmoore
President, Saskatchewan Union of Nurses (SUN)

Provincial View
Tracy Zambory

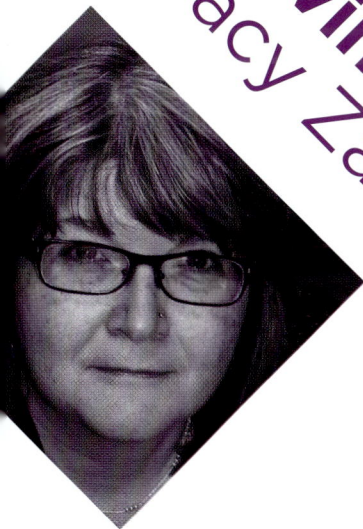

Chapter 10

Long-term care facilities in Saskatchewan are often operating with minimal or even no registered nurse staff. Employers are replacing RNs with other health care providers, which puts into question whether they are fulfilling their legal obligations, says Tracy Zambory, an RN with 25 years of experience nursing in long-term care.

"In fact it would appear that the employers are abandoning long-term care... they have done an abysmal job of retaining and recruiting RNs in long-term care because their focus has been to keep acute care fully staffed. Long-term care is a distant second."

A 2008 report from the Saskatchewan Union of Nurses noted that, despite requirements, a significant proportion of facilities had no RNs on evening and night shifts.

Yet research shows that when RNs are removed, morbidity and mortality rise, says Zambory. "The number of urinary tract infections rises exponentially... and the same for pressure ulcers." Already, complications are on the rise in Saskatchewan facilities, she says.

Disturbingly, this bid to reduce the presence of RNs in long-term care is happening at a time when in Saskatchewan, and indeed everywhere else in Canada, residents are sicker than in the past, with more disease processes and "lots of co-morbidity," she explains.

Saskatchewan's Patient First Review has called for an overhaul of long-term care, but Zambory says she has seen very little regarding this 'overhaul,' although there has been talk of changes to models of care — how care is given and which health care provider is responsible for what. Previously, some long-term care facilities adopted the Eden model. The premise of this model is to make a more home-like atmosphere, with a relaxed breakfast and sleep in. It all sounds romantic but it doesn't work. These are residents with complex care needs which require an RNs attention. This model "virtually removes the RN" from care, she says.

In rural Saskatchewan, acute and chronic care hospitals are closing beds and many of the incentive programs for retaining and recruiting RNs have stopped. Cash incentives were drastically cut in the March 2010 budget.

Meanwhile, rural residents who need long-term care don't necessarily get placed in their home community. "They do try to keep you within 100 kilometres, [but] it can take months or years to get back to your home community where, if it's a small community, there may be only a 40-bed facility." For home care in rural Saskatchewan, RNs have a huge area to cover and they are only allotted a very short amount of time for each client, she says.

A "huge loss" was the cancellation of the Representative Workforce Initiative which was designed to get more First Nations into the workplace and educate existing staff to ensure a smooth transition. "It was such an incredible step backwards," says Zambory, who explains that negotiators had managed to get collective agreements to include opportunities for staff to take representative workforce training.

Asked what she thinks could improve the situation, Zambory stressed the need for more education of the public and governments about what is happening in long-term care. "People don't get concerned until they are personally affected. My hope is that a lot of education can happen, and that the rising up of the people will turn the tide so long-term care is put on the radar and gets the respect it deserves."

What You Told Us About Long-Term Care: A Report From the Saskatchewan Union of Nurses to its Members

In a 2008 report, the Saskatchewan Union of Nurses observed that their members identified (through survey research) a significant erosion of care for the residents of long-term care facilities as well as workloads that are overwhelming and unmanageable.

One of the first issues identified in the report was that nurses feel that they do not have enough time to provide direct care and physical assessments that are required in order to observe the changes in residents' physical and mental health — leaving patients at risk for prolonged hospitalization and for increased personal and social care.

Wallace, M. (2003). *What You Told Us About Long-Term Care: A Report From the Saskatchewan Union of Nurses to its Members.*

Several years ago, the Manitoba Nurses Union conducted a comprehensive study of long-term care in Manitoba. The ensuing report concluded that while Manitoba had seen improvements over the preceding five years and had the highest ratio of long-term care beds to population in Canada, our system failed to meet acceptable standards in several areas. Resident acuity and mental health issues had increased, but staffing models and facility standards had not adapted. A government/union/employer committee was created to study staffing guidelines and make recommendations. The result was the establishment of 3.6 care hours per patient. Government allocated increased funds for long-term care, which were dispersed in the first year but frozen as the economy worsened. Long-term care must be a priority. Nurses now care for patients who require one-to-one care, while being responsible for 75-100 patients on a shift. We care for patients with Alzheimer's, post-operative patients, dementia patients, frail elderly, wanderers and the young disabled. This creates potentially dangerous situations for nurses and patients. Incidents of assault are common. Nurses struggle to provide care in a system that is desperately in need of more resources.

Sandi Mowat
President, Manitoba Nurses Union (MNU)

Provincial View
Judy Robertson

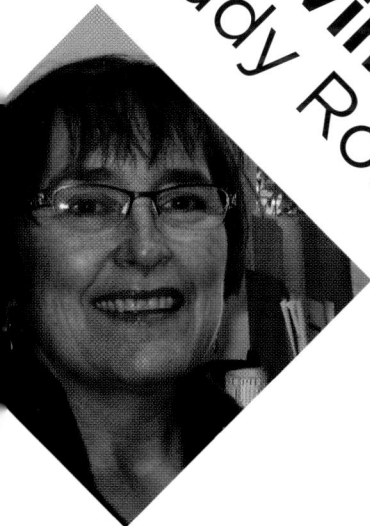

Chapter 11

High rates of dementia among residents in long-term residential care pose challenges that make it vital to employ skilled and passionate nursing staff, says Judy Robertson of Winnipeg, Manitoba.

And facility redesign should be on the agenda, because the calling-out behaviours associated with dementia are disruptive in the long halls and multi-bed rooms that characterize so many current facilities, she says.

"The more people, the noisier, and the noisier it is, the more those people become agitated. We need smaller units."

The Manitoba Centre for Health Policy identified that 65% of residents in long-term care have some form of dementia, but Robertson, a clinical nurse specialist, says in her experience rates are higher, in the range of 80%.

"We try to keep people out of nursing homes," and so when they are admitted, they need more intense care, she says.

But nurses don't graduate clamouring to come to work in long-term care, and "we are still struggling to attract nurses. Maybe we have to change the educational experience and recognize that caring for the elderly is a specialty that requires a great deal of skill and education. The work is very complex and challenging and not easy."

While the care needs of residents have increased, so have the demands for documentation. As a result, nurses spend a great deal of time with electronic assessment tools and care-planning software. "There are demands for the health care system to be more accountable — for example, to document why and when you use a restraint — and these are all goods things that we should be doing. But it really does impact on the workload of nurses and their ability to provide care."

While the province of Manitoba recognized the need to improve staffing ratios and allocated some money for this in 2010, the amount was frozen for 2011. "Under the plans, it would be better, but it would still not be great, because the care needs are so high. If we truly want residents to have a good quality of life, and the staff to feel good about their work, we are going to have to dedicate more money to long-term care."

A greater emphasis on permanent assignment models, in which the same staff work with the same resident day in and day out, makes sense to Robertson. Because of the lack of research into long-term care, it's not entirely clear whether this approach is better than the more common model of rotating staff from unit to unit. "But we are slowly getting more evidence that shows you will diminish issues related to behaviour if you have consistent staffing because you get to know that person intimately and what causes them to be happy and content, and you can anticipate their needs better. Happier residents mean happier staff."

Robertson would like to see much more talk about the future of long-term care, person-centred care, the physical environment and consistent staffing. "A lot of this boils down to money, and what we can afford and what we value. We may not get all we want, but hopefully by the time I get there it will be a lot better than it is now."

Long-Term Care in Manitoba

A 2006 report by the Manitoba Nurses Union examined long-term care in Manitoba.
It found:

- 84% of nurses working in a non-profit facility would recommend their facility to a family member, compared to 67% of nurses in for-profit facilities.
- 56% of nurses in non-profit facilities rated supplies as "good" or "excellent," compared to 40% of those in for-profit facilities.
- By every measure (hip fractures, non-hip fractures, accidental falls, skin ulcers, respiratory infections and fluid/electrolyte imbalances), for-profit facilities reported higher average rates of negative events than non-profit facilities.
- Nurses reported over 300 incidents in 2005 where "insufficient staff" was a factor.
- Almost 20% of nurses reported a resident-nurse ratio of greater than 80:1 on night shifts.

The report provides a number of concrete recommendations to address five key issues:

1) Facility standards
2) Staffing guidelines
3) Workplace violence
4) Recruitment and retention
5) Public accountability

Manitoba Nurses Union. (2006). *Long-Term Care in Manitoba.* Winnipeg: Author. Retrieved from:
http://www.manitobanurses.ca/briefs-reports/
long-term-care-in-manitoba.html

The Ontario hospital system rushes patients out the door far earlier in their recoveries. The home care system is underfunded and understaffed, unable to provide the kind of care/support needed to give clients the option to stay safely in their own homes. A recent trend in Ontario is to admit "rehabilitation" patients or patients on a wait list for long-term care into a for-profit retirement home. These facilities may have home care support services; may (but not likely) be staffed with an RN around the clock; and may represent an enormous financial burden. Currently a patient admitted to a long-term care home in Ontario will typically have multiple diagnoses and medications and require multiple medical treatments and/or behavioural therapies for mental illness or dementia. These homes have not increased the number of hours of registered nursing care per day even though Ontario has one of the lowest-staffed long-term care systems in the country. Seniors should not be forced to live in a long-term care home (perhaps at considerable distance) because it is cheaper to provide understaffed institutional care. Nurses and other care providers in long-term care should be paid and respected as are their hospital counterparts.

Linda Haslam-Stroud
President, Ontario Nurses' Association (ONA)

Provincial View
Beverly Mathers

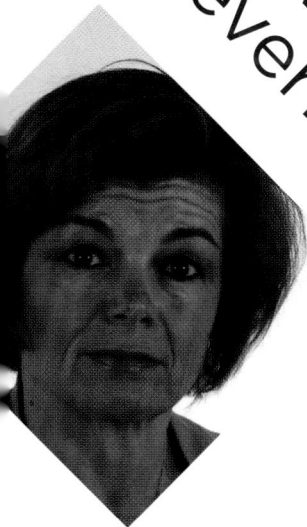

Chapter 12

The pressure to discharge patients from hospital, combined with inadequate levels of home care, have led to dramatic changes in the care needs of older Ontarians who are admitted to long-term care, says Beverly Mathers, RN, BA, MA.

"Years ago, a typical admission would be the frail granny who was at home and maybe forgot to eat and might be malnourished, or maybe forgot and left the stove on. Today residents have at least two diagnoses, and many have between three and five. On average, they are taking eight medications per day, and they may be getting multiple treatments — dialysis, tube feeding, intravenous — a myriad of treatments that would never have been provided in long-term care in the past."

But the skills and ratio of staff have not kept pace with changes. "If anything, staff are less skilled — there are more unregulated workers than we have ever had in the past and fewer registered nurses."

Other political changes have increased the risks for elderly residents. Policies of deinstitutionalization have led to a situation where many individuals who are now placed in long-term care facilities would, in the past, have lived in psychiatric hospitals or developmental centres. These residents "are often ambulatory with unpredictable behaviour and yet they are comingled with the frail elderly" thus posing significant risks to other residents and to staff.

Ontario recently enacted legislation that consolidates the previous "hodgepodge" of acts, regulations and policies that governed different types of long-term care in the province. However, despite the recommendations of a 2001 government-commissioned report and a 2005 report from a coroner's inquest into nursing home deaths, the province did not set minimum hours of care per resident, Mathers says. The legislation does stipulate that each and every long-term care home should have one registered nurse on duty around the clock. However, this requirement is "not bad if the home has 60 beds, but horrendous if it has 300 beds." And larger facilities are more common. More than 50% of long-term care beds in Ontario are in for-profit facilities — the highest proportion of any province — and because of economies of scale, there is "very little investment" in facilities with fewer than 100 beds, Mathers notes.

Ontario's new legislation calls for a more home-like atmosphere, including changes such as spreading meal times over a longer period. "It's a great thing for residents. If you are 79 years old and never were a morning person, do you really want to be up at breakfast at 7:30?"

But Mathers warns that without adequate staffing and training, the requirement to create a more home-like environment "amounts to useless words on a piece of paper." For instance, adequate staffing is particularly important for continence care since being continent "is the last shred of dignity everyone has and, to keep it, residents need toileting regularly." Time and workload pressures on staff mean residents who need help to get to the toilet are often put in diapers for the sake of convenience.

Meanwhile, keeping staff in long-term care in Ontario is "really a struggle." Nurses' salary and benefits are higher in Ontario hospitals and wage competition means a lot of long-term care facilities just cannot recruit. "We can't get new young nurses in — or if we do, they might work three or five shifts before realizing they can make more money, get more benefits, and have more support in hospitals. So we have a very senior workforce, many of whom are preparing to retire," Mathers explains. Ontario's 2007 Aging at Home Strategy promised to "transform community health care services so that seniors can live healthy, independent lives in their own homes." But despite this promise of enhanced service, Mathers says, the reality looks different. The Community Care Access Centres, with a mandate to organize home care in local areas, "have deficits, wait lists for services, and there is a shortage of service providers, and that does complicate things... we promised to provide the services to keep people at home, but we can't fulfil that promise."

"It really is absolutely devastating how we are treating our seniors," Mathers concludes.

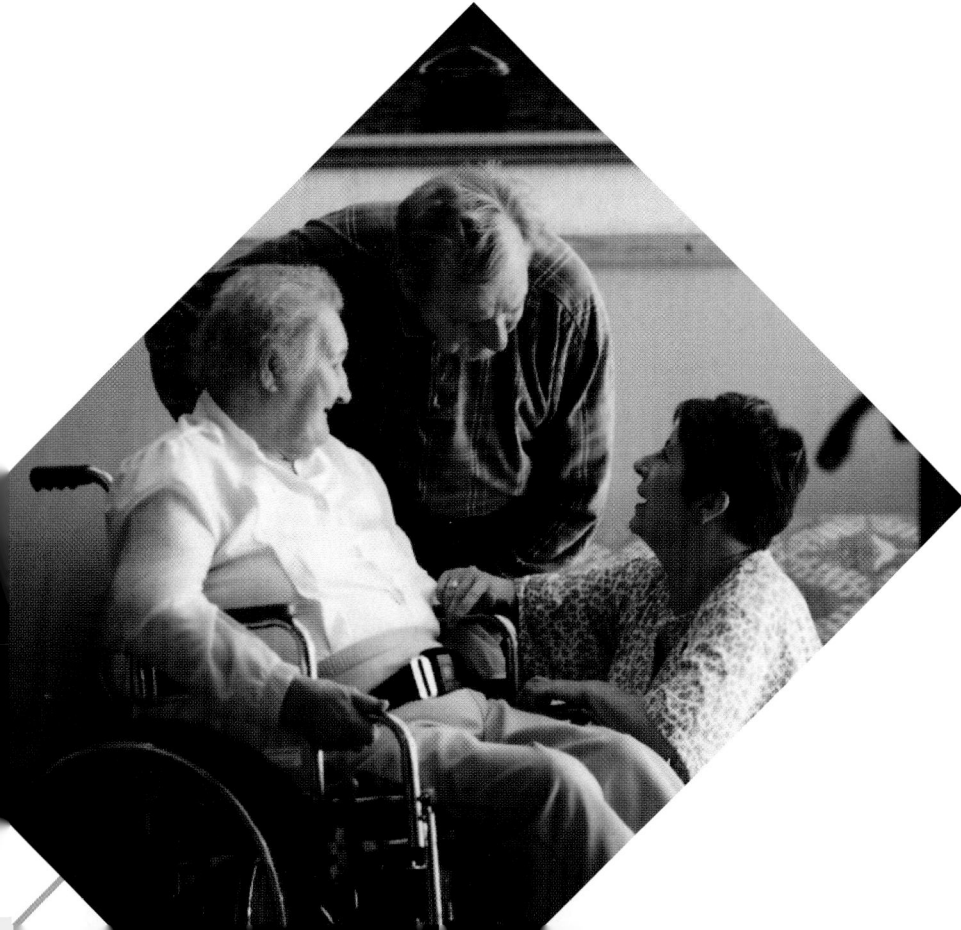

Home Care, Continuing Care and Medicare: A Canadian Model or Innovative Models for Canadians?

"...access to home care is inequitable in Canada. Financing mechanisms should improve integration of care, not increase barriers between medical, hospital and social care."

Béland, F. & Bergman, H. (2000). Home Care, Continuing Care and Medicare: A Canadian Model or Innovative Models for Canadians? *HealthcarePapers* 1(4): 38-45.

Research to Action

A multi-year, multi-jurisdictional applied research project was developed by CFNU in 2008. With support from Health Canada, this series of ten pilot projects is known as Research to Action: Applied Workplace Solutions for Nurses (RTA).

Newfoundland and Labrador now has the oldest demographic in Canada but the capacity for gerontological care was not keeping pace due to a lack of care personnel, particularly nurses.

It is often harder to recruit and retain RNs in the long-term care (LTC) sector than in acute settings. Recognizing this, among other issues, the Newfoundland & Labrador Nurses' Union, the provincial Department of Health, and Central Regional Health Authority proposed the adoption of an 80/20 RN staffing model where nurses spend 80% of their time in direct patient care and 20% in professional development and mentoring.

Carmelite House was chosen as the implementation site for the project. The 64-bed LTC facility is located in Grand Falls-Windsor, a town of about 15,000 in the Newfoundland interior. Project objectives include:

- Providing time for RNs to develop leadership and clinical skills, engage in work-related activities, and enhance a resident-centered environment.
- Enhancing the profile of LTC as a desired workplace choice and increasing the RN retention rates in LTC facilities.

More information about this project and others that address issues in LTC can be found at: http://www.thinknursing.ca/RTA

In the mid 90s, the Quebec government imposed the "shift to ambulatory care."
The objective was to treat and maintain patients in their communities. The required
investment in home care did not follow. Fifteen years later, according to the Canadian
Institute for Health Information (CIHI), Quebec remains among the lowest when it
comes to dedicating funding to home support. Service integration projects, such as
SIPA (Services intégrés pour personnes âgées — Research Program on Integrated
Services for the Elderly), were abandoned due to a lack of funding. Consequently, the
Quebec government relies on families and informal caregivers for numerous services.
Patients who have lost their independence or are suffering from chronic diseases,
many of whom have no family doctor, have to go to hospital emergency departments,
creating recurring overflows. This creates gaps in the continuity of care provided by
professionals who are missing pertinent information about the patient's treatment or
general knowledge of the patients to treat them adequately.

Régine Laurent
President, Fédération interprofessionnelle de la santé du Québec (FIQ)

Provincial View
François Béland

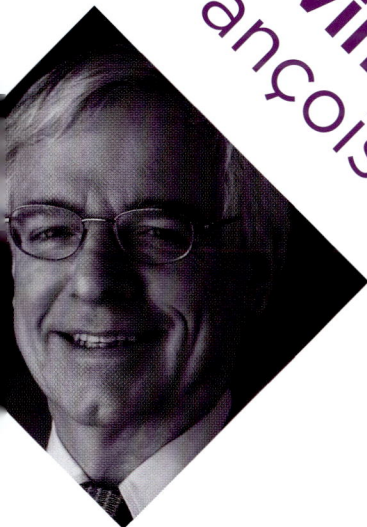

Chapter 13

Continuing care for the elderly is riddled with perverse financial incentives that force people who could be supported at home into institutions, and attempts to address this in Quebec have faced challenges, says François Béland.

For example, when an elderly person needs home care services that cost in the range of $15,000 to $20,000 a year, they usually have a condition that makes them eligible for a nursing home, says Béland, a professor of health administration at the Université de Montréal Faculty of Medicine. "So from the point of view of home care services, because of their own budget concerns, this person should be institutionalized."

But at about $50,000 a year, the cost for a person to be a resident in a nursing home is more than twice that of keeping them at home, where they may well prefer to stay. "It's all public money, so globally this is a waste of public money… but no one in the system can really think of it this way," he says.

Elderly Canadians who need care likely see hospital care, long-term care, and home care as all being part of one system. But in fact there is no real system, and the latter two are not part of the *Canada Health Act,* which means access to them "is not guaranteed and it will be quite partial."

Former Quebec Health Minister Philippe Couillard tried to address some of this system fragmentation in 2004 with the integration, at the local level, of Centres locaux de services communautaires (CLSCs), nursing homes, and hospitals into Centres de santé et de services sociaux (CSSS).

The change was "an effort to look globally at the sector, instead of looking at bits and pieces. But it seems to be very, very different in different settings, in some CSSSs it's working, and in some others it isn't. For example, budgets are not flowing easily from nursing homes to home, social, and health care programs."

As well, the enormous energy that was put into implementing the reform meant that some well-functioning organizations that were merged have paid the price of "energy going to the merger rather than to delivering the services."

In Béland's view, the Couillard reform "was trying to merge the organizations so there would be fluidity in the system, but this was all theoretical, and done from the point of view of reforming the structure of the system and not in terms of the clinical model."

A change in the clinical model would "allow people to have access to the best services at the least cost." However, making this change happen would mean adjusting financial incentives and negotiating with professional organizations around the organization of care — things that politicians are loath to do.

Many European countries have introduced what they call the fifth pillar of social security, which is insurance for long-term care. "Coverage is quite different in different countries, the way they are doing it, whether it is merged or not with health care system. But at least they have looked into long-term care as a global system."

In Quebec, the 2001 report of the Clair Commission proposed European style social security funding for long-term care for the elderly. "I may not agree with it, but at least there has been some thinking" on the issue, says Béland.

Béland would like to see universal coverage of long-term care, including home care. "People would have to make some contribution — I have no objection to people paying for room and board in public nursing homes, adjusted to their income — but the care component, the medical and social care component, should be fully covered."

Guaranteeing Access: Meeting the Challenges of Equity, Efficiency and Quality

A report from Québec identifies a need to "adopt service-provision methods that are firmly oriented towards supporting people in the community, particularly those in need of long-term care and the most vulnerable members of society."

Specifically, "the health and social services system must adapt, and must adopt practices and technologies that will respond better to changes in the population's needs."

It acknowledges a need to "make use of all available skills by focusing on optimal sharing of tasks, particularly between nurses and physicians; and adopt service-provision modes oriented towards supporting people in the community, particularly for those with a permanent incapacity and those for whom accommodation environments must be diversified and the various home-support programs reviewed."

Gouvernement du Québec (2006). *Guaranteeing Access: Meeting the Challenges of Equity, Efficiency and Quality: Consultation document.* La Direction des communications du ministère de la Santé et des Services sociaux. Retrieved from: http://publications.msss.gouv.qc.ca/acrobat/f/documentation/2005/05-721-01A.pdf

As the number of seniors in our province increases, so too will the demand for long-term care services. Although the crunch felt by demographic changes will not be fully felt until the baby boomers are in their seventies, we must start planning now. NBNU realizes that as the aging population increases, the population will decrease because of the trend towards smaller families. This fiscal reality should be handled through adjustments to a number of programs, the first being an increase in the long-term care bed capacity, which would not only relieve beds presently used in hospitals for those on long-term care wait lists, it would also improve the quality of life for many seniors. Those waiting for long-term care placement in hospitals have limits on the kind of care they can receive. Specialized care that would be provided in a nursing home is not available and the setting in an acute care facility is inappropriate for someone waiting for long-term care. We must always remember that a society will be judged on the basis of how it treats its weakest and most vulnerable citizens.

Marilyn Quinn
President, New Brunswick Nurses Union (NBNU)

Provincial View
Violet Budd

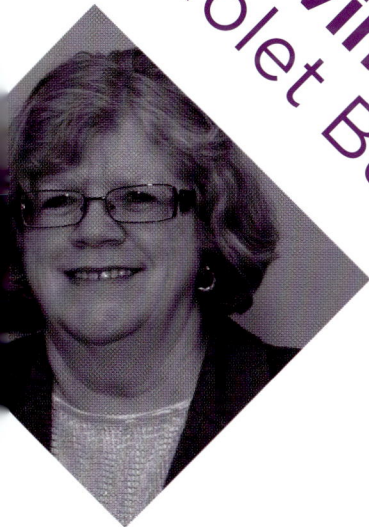

Chapter 14

A 2007 report by the Canadian Institute for Health Information (Drug Claims by Seniors: An Analysis Focusing on Potentially Inappropriate Medication Use, 2000 to 2006) indicates that 8-12% of seniors in Alberta, Saskatchewan, Manitoba and New Brunswick had a long-term prescription for a high-risk drug on the Beer's List. The Beer's list identifies drugs that are potentially inappropriate to prescribe to seniors due to an elevated risk of adverse effects.

As a nurse in the geriatric department of a large hospital, Violet Budd sees patients admitted from both the community and nursing homes because of inadequate availability of resources to provide quality care.

Older people who live at home and are at risk "don't get seen and assessed fast enough. We often get patients admitted because they didn't get the care or services that they need." The system is "just not efficient enough," Budd concludes.

Older people who live in the community often "don't know how to get help other than to go to hospital, unless they are linked up with a seniors' group or health charity." Meanwhile, their health may have deteriorated when all they needed to maintain independence was "two or three hours a day of help — for someone to help with personal care, house cleaning, shopping, etc."

But for this type of basic home support service, there is a long wait list to get the necessary social worker assessment, and for those deemed eligible for help, it is provided on a means-tested co-pay basis, she says.

As for pressure areas, Budd says some of the problem comes down to a lack of education. There are various causes of skin breakdown including immobility, lack of pressure relief and malnutrition. "Not everyone understands the importance of nutrition. You can't maintain your tissue without adequate protein and calories, and sometimes health care providers — never mind untrained people — don't know that. But if you don't eat, and your blood counts are low, you really can't heal yourself, so pressure sores happen because a person is too thin or not getting what they need to live."

But Budd also says the number of care hours per person in the nursing homes is insufficient. A decade or more ago, many nursing home residents were up and active and many of them had their own cars in the parking lot. Now, it is a different world: "When I see patients who go from hospital to nursing homes, a lot are in wheelchairs, need mechanical lifts to get in and out of bed. They can maybe wash their face and hands but the rest is provided care. Some need to be fed. A lot need thickened liquids because their gag reflex is gone. There are catheters, and tube feeding, and they are starting to expect homes to take people with tracheotomies and breathing tubes."

Budd says she hears "horror stories" from nurses who work in the nursing homes about the difficulties the staff are dealing with. "You think, 'My God, I hope I never have to go there or put my family there.' And it's not the staff's fault. It is just that there isn't the staff that there should be."

The goal at her geriatric service ward is to "get people back to their previous level of functioning. So if there was an event at home, we start working with them to find out, for example, the reason for a fall." Medications — multiple medications and drug interactions — are often involved. "A lot of seniors haven't had a good medication review for a long time and they come in with multiple prescriptions." Patients who have undergone surgery are often taking a lot of painkillers and sedatives. "Quite often they will be considered to have dementia when actually it is delirium caused by medications and anaesthesia. Often when an elderly person gets the same dose for pain as a young person, it causes major confusion and disorientation. The three Ds — dementia, delirium and depression — have some of the same presentations."

When people are housebound, especially in winter, a home visit can be made for drawing blood or dressing a wound. That is possible because of New Brunswick's Extra-Mural Program. But at many seniors' apartments, there is a charge for services such as help with insulin and medications, says Budd. "If you are at home and need help with your insulin, it is part of EMP [Extra-Mural Program], so why shouldn't it be covered elsewhere?" In her view, all medical care needs should be covered by the provincial medicare plan.

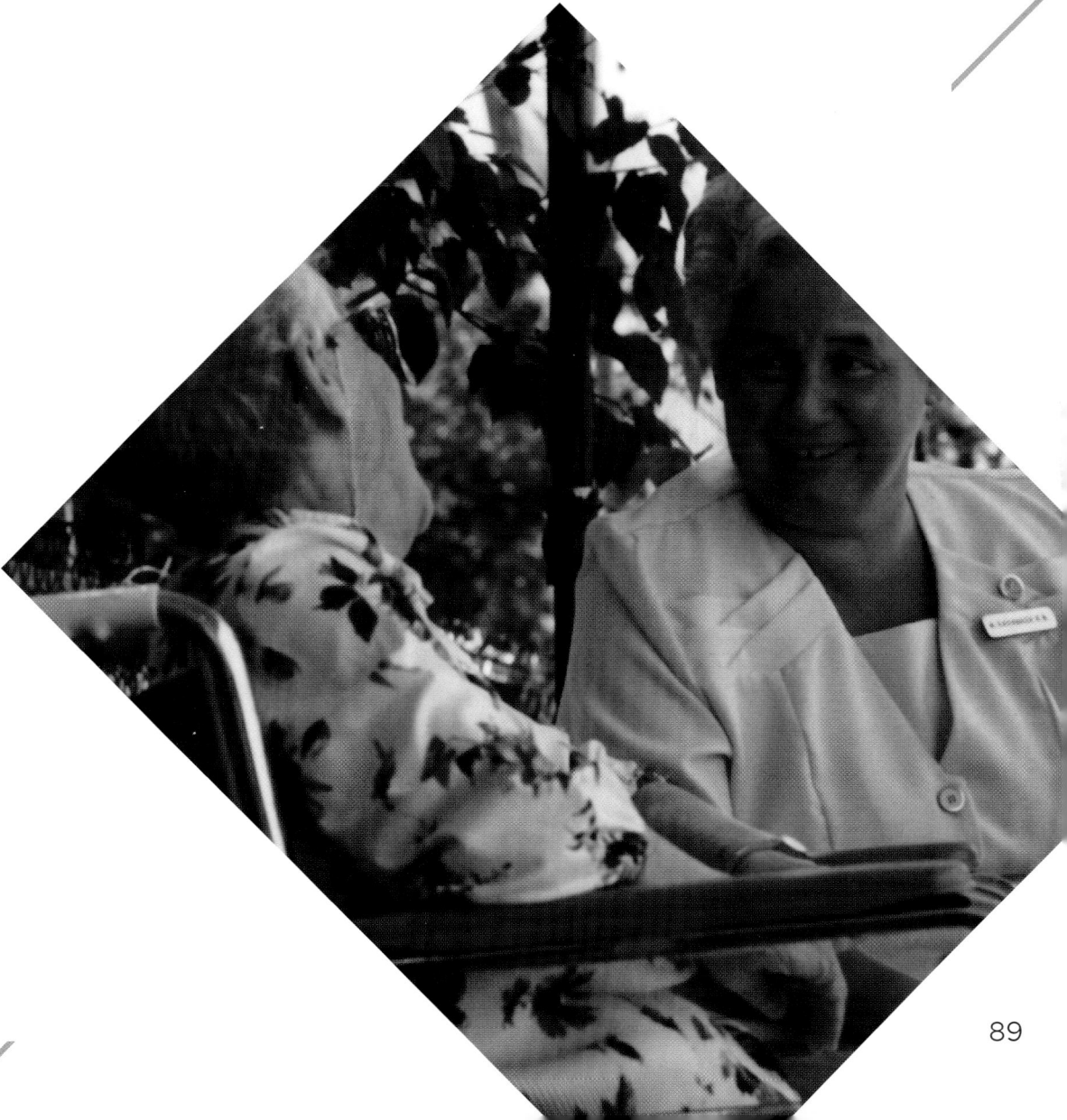

First Nations Action Plan on Continuing Care

"First Nations peoples' health is in crisis. The demand for institutional and related continuing care services for First Nations will grow rapidly over the next several decades due to increases in the number of First Nation members aged 55 and older. The 55-64-year age group will increase by 236% and the 65+ age group will increase by 229% in this period. There will be 57,000 more First Nations members aged 65 and older in 2021."

"The main ongoing gaps are perceived to be palliative care, rehabilitative care, respite care and mental health services."

The First Nations and Inuit Home and Community Care program addressed some of the more significant gaps in services (including case management, nursing care and personal care) but specifically excludes the construction of institutional long-term care facilities and the delivery of institutional long-term care services. This is a critical gap as it limits access to culturally appropriate services.

"First Nations have grave concerns over the increasing number of Elders who are being placed in facilities outside their communities because of the current lack of opportunity to develop community-based, culturally appropriate alternatives to provincial institutional care, such as group homes, foster care, adult day care or more intensive enhanced in-home care services. First Nations feel isolated in provincial facilities and are often situated long distances from their families. This has a detrimental effect on their health and quality of life."

Assembly of First Nations. (2005). *First Nations Action Plan on Continuing Care.* Retrieved from:
http://64.26.129.156/cmslib/general/CCAP.pdf

Long-term care facilities in Nova Scotia are challenged by underfunding, limited resources and overwhelmed front-line staff, yet the case for improving palliative care in nursing homes is strong. The majority of Canada's elderly die in hospitals or long-term care facilities. Currently, many palliative level long-term care residents with multiple chronic conditions undergo frequent transitions between the nursing home and emergency or hospital wards. Increased hospitalizations expose the resident to higher risk. Hospitalized residents more frequently experience serious problems such as medication errors, falls, difficulty with new care plans and unfamiliar staff and settings.

The erosion of licensed, registered staff has left long-term care woefully inadequate to provide optimal palliative care, off-loading this on to an overextended acute care system. An increase in the numbers of professional regulated staff along with educational opportunities would reduce costs by decreasing hospital admissions. Improving the quality of palliative care in long-term care will require systematic and cultural change done in collaborative partnerships with stakeholders at all levels.

Janet Hazelton
President, Nova Scotia Nurses' Union (NSNU)

Provincial View
Doreen Charman

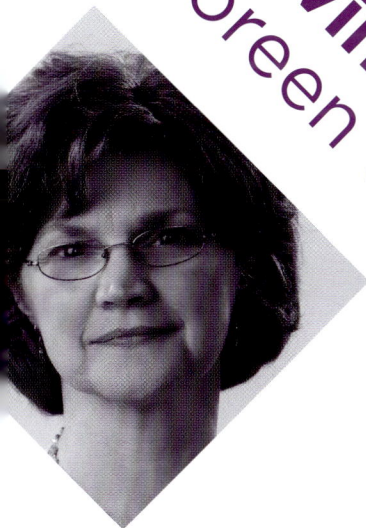

Chapter 15

Residents are more likely to die in their nursing home beds these days because of the greater availability of palliative care, says Doreen Charman, a Nova Scotia nurse with more than two decades of experience in long-term care.

It's a positive development for residents, but comes at a cost of staff, she says.

"In the past, people often died on stretchers all alone in emergency rooms instead of in their own bed in a nursing home, with proper care from people who know them, are attached, and often love them. We try very hard, when there has been a change in condition, to get the doctors in to do an assessment and diagnosis and set down a care plan rather than call an ambulance."

The change has been brought on partly because of hospitals' lack of capacity and mostly by compassion, she says. "But all this adds to the stress of working in the homes. I think we do palliative care extremely well, but it is at a cost to staff. It's not funded at the same levels as hospital palliative units — absolutely not, you don't get bells and whistles. But you do get the compassion and caring and we do the best we can with what we've got and for the most part we do a good job."

Still, staffing is an issue. Shortages are "constant and ongoing. It's been going on for decades, but it is worse. There is more competition for human resources."

Nova Scotia has the highest proportion of people over 65 years old in the country — which means both greater needs and an aging workforce. Charman herself plans to retire in the near future, in part so she can be available to help care for her elderly mother.

Meanwhile, with upgrades and expansions, the number of nursing home beds in the province has increased in the past couple of years, "which heats up the battle for staff." For example, there is a shortage of registered nurses and, because those in long-term care have been formally trained to deal with seniors, "acute care is scooping them up."

Staffing issues, the greater care needs of residents, and budget concerns have all contributed to another noteworthy change that Charman has observed — the downloading of responsibility onto families for the needs of nursing home residents.

"Before we were more paternalistic in our care: we made appointments for residents, arranged attendants and arranged for them to get there. Now, if you are going to see an eye doctor, are you willing to pay for transportation? There is always help, some subsidy available, but definitely there is more responsibility on families. The family still needs to make decisions, and if there is an acute process, there are costs involved."

As for home care, Charman knows from personal experience that it is limited. "My mother, who is 87, is in her home and has had a couple of bad falls in the past year with fractures. We have been able to get care in place for her, but the bottom line is once she no longer needs the VON nursing care related to an acute process — which is an hour in the morning and an hour in the evening — then she will be alone in the house a lot."

And Charman also wonders about her own future. "I firmly believe in the public good, and we need to take care of our population as it ages. It is all well and good to say we have to take care of ourselves, but most of us will outlive our money. Where will my friends and I be in 15 or 20 years? We need to brainstorm and put our heads together. How will we access and provide the care that is needed?"

For-Profit Versus Not-For Profit Delivery of Long-Term Care

"About 60% and 30% of all publicly funded long-term care beds in Ontario and British Columbia respectively are in for-profit institutions."

"....we are beginning to acquire evidence from Canadian data that public investment in not-for profit, rather than for-profit, delivery of long-term care results in more staffing and improved care outcomes for residents. This information is essential to planners as they make decisions about long-term care."

McGrail, K., McGregor, M., Cohen, M., Tate, R. & Ronald, L. (2007). For-Profit Versus Not-For-Profit Delivery of Long-Term Care. *Canadian Medical Association Journal,* 176(1), 57-58.

It is disturbing that the delivery methods of health care for our most senior and fragile citizens are being looked at as a means to achieve cost savings through reductions in nursing staff. Our members who work in long-term care facilities are experienced and knowledgeable health care professionals in their specialty. They are acutely aware of the benefits derived by long-term care residents when professional caregivers have the opportunity to provide direct patient care. Conversely, they are also aware of how the quality of care is negatively impacted when the number of registered nurses at the bedside is reduced. The employer is ignoring evidence-based research that supports what our members already know and experience at the bedside.

Long-term care facilities are not merely "end-of-life" institutions. Some residents spend many years in these facilities. They continue to depend upon the expertise RNs offer in order to maintain their health and experience enjoyment in their lives. We believe the latest move to reduce front-line long-term care RNs is a step backwards for the health and welfare of our seniors.

Mona O'Shea
President, Prince Edward Island Nurses' Union (PEINU)

Provincial View
Doreen Wyand

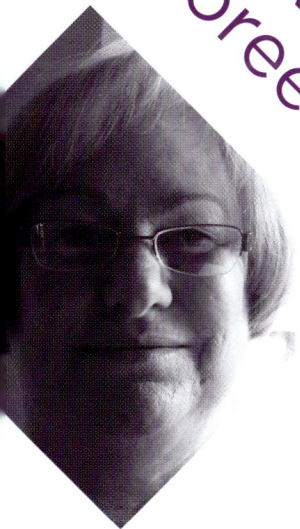

Chapter 16

When an international consultancy firm documented the fact that Prince Edward Island's public nursing homes had higher standards for staffing than other provinces, their advice was clear: lower those standards.

Acting on the 2008 consultants' report, the province is also deleting nursing positions from many facilities, says Doreen Wyand, a nurse with more than 25 years of experience working in a public long-term care facility in PEI.

"It is very, very unpleasant... We can't see the overall picture; they are rolling out pilots in different facilities."

The report stated that "staffing in public manors, which provide 3.69 to 4.25 hours per resident per day, differs from other provinces and should be brought down," she explained.

The decision to lower standards is "nonsense, considering the complexity of care that is now required in our facilities. Many of the elderly, frail with comorbidities, who are coming into nursing homes aren't what you would consider stable. We are staffed to the bare bones as it is."

Indeed, the level of care needs of residents is such that the house doctor at Wyand's facility says staff is providing "acute care for the elderly."

"Inconsistent with emerging research and trends," is how Wyand says the consultants labelled PEI's ratio of long-term beds to population. The report also set targets such as how quickly beds should be filled. "So you have a resident that you have grown close to, that you see day after day, they become like a family to you. If you read this report, you have to get their room cleared out and fill that bed tomorrow. To a lot of staff it becomes really disrespectful to the person."

Wyand marvels at the people in the community who are looking after relatives. "The report says we should look at providing more home-based care, but I don't think that has changed. The majority of care is still done by the informal caregiver."

There are three respite care beds in the facility where Wyand works and they are filled almost all the time. "I look at the husband, wife, son or daughter bringing in their relative, and shake my head and wonder — how in the world are they looking after them at home. In some instances they have many complex care needs."

When new residents are admitted, they are often taking numerous medications and may not know why they are taking them. "It becomes quite apparent sometimes that they were put on meds years ago, for example when they might have had high blood pressure, but were left on even if their blood pressure is now fine." Often they have had problems with sleep and are taking medications. "When they come into our facility, we quickly try to decrease and then stop sleeping meds. It increases the risks of falls when they take sedatives. But many residents now have been taking meds for a long time and are adamant that they need them."

Sparked by concern about the number of medications that residents were taking, Wyand and colleagues convinced their employer to have a provincial pharmacist review the situation. "I would fax her four or five med sheets each day, and she would do a write-up, noting where there could be an interaction, and make recommendations." The facility's house doctor came to trust the pharmacist's opinion.

Unfortunately, the innovation was short-lived and the home no longer has the services of a consulting pharmacist.

Providing Care and Support For an Aging Population: Briefing Notes on Key Policy Issues

"Reducing resources for long-term home care and home support may bring about an ever-increasing cost spiral as people in need put more pressure on hospital beds and residential care beds — leading to more demands for budget increases from hospitals."

"Long-term home care may in fact be an important part of the solution to making our overall health care system more efficient and effective, and enhancing its value for money."

Hollander, M., Chappell, N., Prince, M. & Shapiro, E. (2007). Providing Care and Support For an Aging Population: Briefing Notes on Key Policy Issues. *Healthcare Quarterly* 10(3): 34-45.

Making it possible for people to live in the comfort and familiarity of their homes is central to the continuum of care. But to truly support this approach, we must drastically improve the supports provided to home care workers and, in particular, to family members caring for loved ones.

A recent study by the Canadian Institute for Health Information indicates that 98% of seniors receiving home care had an informal caregiver at home, like a spouse or adult, and that one in six are in distress and at risk of burnout. For many, it is emotionally, physically and financially draining.

We need to stand up for these caregivers and ease the challenges they face every day. This means ensuring they have proper training and resources, adequate financial support and respite care so they have time to rest and recharge.

Debbie Forward
President, Newfoundland and Labrador Nurses' Union (NLNU)

Provincial View
Kathleen Connors

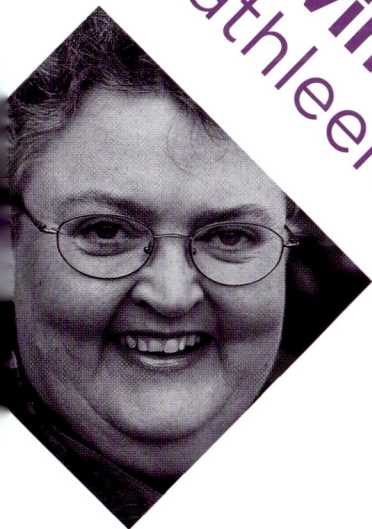

Chapter 17

The lack of training requirements for paid home care workers, their scarcity in rural areas, and the shortage of support for unpaid family caregivers are key concerns in Newfoundland and Labrador where the collapse of the fishery has led sons and daughters to leave the province to find work.

"Many seniors are truly alone in a province where traditionally families have borne the caregiving responsibility," says Kathleen Connors, a retired nurse and member of a provincial network that advocates around issues related to aging. "And rural seniors are particularly disadvantaged." There's a long list of caregiving agencies in the city of St. John's, but there may be no caregivers in smaller communities and rural areas, she notes.

If the province had a proper, publicly funded home care and home support program, seniors could enjoy quality of care while remaining in the comfort of their own homes and communities, says Connors, a past president of the Canadian Federation of Nurses Unions and chair of the Canadian Health Coalition, who now lives in Pouch Cove.

But too often, seniors in small and rural communities who need help end up having to move to personal care homes or nursing homes outside their home communities. "And when you remove people from their social support network, from their friends and family, it can be psychologically and emotionally devastating for them."

Quality of care is also an issue. All that's necessary to become a home support worker in the province is "a certificate of conduct, which is police clearance, and a first aid course," Connors explains. What's needed is policies and standards that are consistent around the province with consequences for individuals and agencies that don't comply.

Connors said her advocacy network "talked to one woman who went from being a fish plant worker to home support, and it absolutely frightened her. Without the training, people are reluctant — they don't want to harm the people they care for."

The government does have an excellent curriculum for personal care worker training, but fees for the 20-week course offered almost exclusively in private colleges range from $5,000-$8,500, she says. "When you graduate you can earn $17.94 an hour in a hospital or nursing home, but only $11.75 in home care. As a result, retaining home care workers is a problem."

In Canada, and indeed in North America, there has been a tendency to "look at dealing with seniors' issues in an institutional framework, rather than in the continuum of care. If we make evidence-based decisions, which we should be doing in health care, the evidence comes down on the side of maintaining people in the community with supports."

Yet what has happened in Canada is a "narrowing" of home care to acute and post-hospital discharge care. "The shift in home care is quite sad. I come from Manitoba and when I graduated in 1972, the home care program was already established and it really was comprehensive. Now my mom needs service in Manitoba, and it has really narrowed. For example, personal support workers are not allowed to do laundry."

When home support workers are unavailable or when seniors can not afford to pay for required services, caregiving often falls to ill-prepared family members. To assist family caregivers, the Seniors' Resource Centre — which receives some core funding from government but remains independent of the provincial government — operates a Caregivers Out of Isolation program. It includes a staff person in the office, with a toll free telephone line, where people can call in with questions and concerns. The staff person deals with a plethora of questions. As well, there is a newsletter and there are networks and support groups around the province. "It is a lifeline for people," Connors explains.

But she says it is important to be careful not to "conscript" people to be unpaid caregivers. To help prepare a report, her advocacy network held focus groups with family care providers. "One woman said her husband expected her to take care of him, but she felt uncomfortable — that she didn't have the knowledge to do things properly, like the rehabilitation exercises or the speech therapy. But she said she felt that she had to do it, that she was conscripted into it by the expectations of her husband and family members. When you tease out how people really feel, you hear things — like the attitude that asking for respite care is a sign of failure."

Connors says that she has come to realize that the emphasis on institutional care for seniors is very North American. "We have looked at dealing with seniors' care issues in an institutional framework, rather than in the context of a continuum of care. In Canada we have looked at the health care system in silos, and the squeaky wheel — to date that means acute care — gets the grease. That means that relatively little attention is paid to the nursing home sector and probably the least attention goes to supportive home care." Canada should be learning from the experience and best practices of countries that have dealt with a large aging population for much longer — countries in the European Union, for example Denmark, she says.

Until there is political will to create a true continuum of services — and especially a publicly funded home care program — families will continue to deal with the silos of personal care homes, nursing homes, and private for-profit home care agencies.

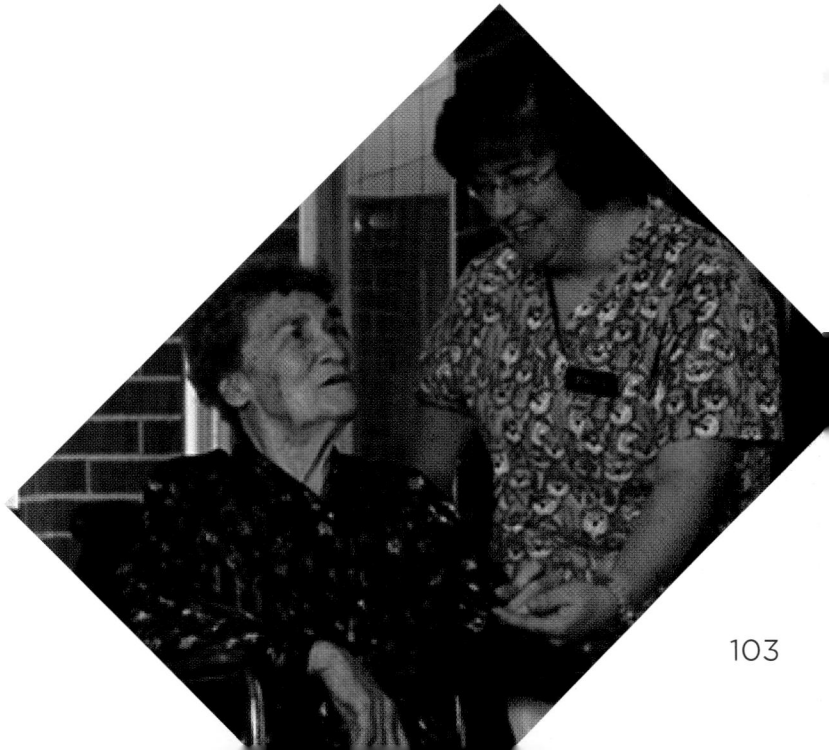

Piecing Together the Continuum of Care

"The pieces of the health care system should fit together in a seamless system of support that maintains or improves the health of seniors and people with disabilities. This is referred to as the continuum of care."

A report by the British Columbia Health Coalition recommends:

- A universal publicly funded and delivered program of improved and expanded home support services;
- Infrastructure to ensure that there are sufficient not-for-profit residential care beds to meet the needs of seniors and people with disabilities; and
- A National Pharmacare Plan.

BC Health Coalition. (2010). *Piecing Together the Continuum of Care: Concerns & Solutions from BC's Health Care Advocates.* Retrieved from: http://healthcoalition.ca/wp-content/uploads/2010/02/BCHC-CC-Piece1.pdf

Jumping on the Alberta Bandwagon

"Forcing seniors, who have paid into the public system for years, to give up almost all their income or spend all their savings to obtain care is a grim betrayal of their generation."

A report written by Wendy Armstrong addresses three myths associated with care for seniors:

Myth #1: People who need LTC services are sophisticated consumers with lots of money.
Reality check: The median income for seniors in Alberta was just over $1,400 per month in 1997.

Myth #2: Shifting the costs and burden of care to family members is costless to society.
Reality check: In fact, shifting sizeable costs and burdens to the family is expensive on personal and societal levels. The stress of constant caregiving can lead to emotional, financial and health breakdowns.

Myth #3: Private health care markets will provide better service and better value for the money.
Reality check: Real competition, affordable prices, and quality controls are difficult to achieve in private health care markets. Further, a fragmented and privatized system is more costly to run than a public system.

Armstrong, W. (2002). *Jumping on the Alberta Bandwagon: Does B.C. Need This Kind of Assisted Living?* Hospital Employees Union, British Columbia. Retrieved from: http://www.albertaconsumers.org/EldercareBC.pdf

Dr. Michael Rachlis

Dr. Michael Rachlis was born in Winnipeg, Manitoba, in 1951 and graduated from the University of Manitoba medical school in 1975. He interned at McMaster University and then practiced family medicine at the South Riverdale Community Health Centre in Toronto for eight years. He completed specialty training in Community Medicine at McMaster and was made a fellow of the Canadian Royal College of Physicians in 1988. Dr. Rachlis practices as a private consultant in health policy analysis. He has consulted to the federal government, all ten provincial governments, and two royal commissions. He is also an associate professor (status only) with the University of Toronto Dalla Lana School of Public Health. In 2010, the University of Manitoba conferred upon Dr. Rachlis a Doctor of Laws in recognition of his service to Canadian health policy. Dr. Rachlis has lectured widely on health care issues. He has been invited to make presentations to committees of the Canadian House of Commons and the Canadian Senate as well as the United States House of Representatives and Senate. He is a frequent media commentator on health policy issues and the author of three national bestsellers about Canada's health care system. In his spare time, Dr. Rachlis enjoys cycling and duplicate bridge.

Continuing Care is an Essential Part of Medicare

Dr. Michael Rachlis

Chapter 18

This book has outlined 17 experts' perceptions of continuing care. This term is used to include both home care and long-term care as it is in Western Canada, although the focus here is on long-term care. The picture isn't pretty. Overall, there has been a Canada-wide deterioration in availability of long-term care beds and home care for patients with chronic care conditions. What is the future for Canadian continuing care?

In fact, these days, one might as well ask, what is the future of medicare and what are the values of equity and justice upon which it relies? I have spoken with tens of thousands of Canadians about our health system. I am more convinced than ever that the vast majority of us see Canada as a place where no family should have to choose between the lack of good care and financial hardship.

Unfortunately, a choir of voices claims that medicare is unsustainable. They allege that continuing care, like pharmacare, is a frill that we can't afford at this time. Neither assertion is true. The first reveals a well-orchestrated campaign to convince Canadians to jettison medicare. The second reveals a profound ignorance about how health systems work.

You don't hear medicare's opponents say that people should choose between paying for groceries or personal care. Rather they claim that medicare is unsustainable now and the boomer silver tsunami will soon finish the job. The diagnosis is typically delivered as firm as fate and as inevitable as tomorrow's sunrise. Their prescriptions are typically public sector cutbacks and more private pay and delivery.

In fact, provincial health spending as a share of our economy (GDP) is only slightly higher than when we were coming out of the last serious recession in the early 1990s. Moreover, health care has only slightly increased its share of provincial budgets, and even these apparent increases are primarily due to the distorting effect of cuts in other program areas rather than absolute increases in health spending.

Finally, aging of the population increases health care costs by less than one percent per year. Population aging is a glacier, not a tsunami. You can't get knocked over by a glacier unless you don't move. The reader can learn more about this issue in *The Sustainability of Medicare,* released by the CFNU in August 2010 at: http://www.nursesunions.ca/news/nurses-urge-first-ministers-negotiate-new-health-accord-2004-accord-set-expire-cfnu-releases-re. Continuing care may not be part of the *Canada Health Act,* but it is an integral part of the health system.

As observed by York University professor Pat Armstrong, continuing care is mainly absent from the *Canada Health Act.* Passed in 1984, the *Canada Health Act* integrates two previous pieces of legislation, the 1957 *Hospital Insurance and Diagnostic Services Act* which covered hospital care and the 1966 *Medical Care Act* which added a national physicians' insurance program.

Justice Emmett Hall's 1964 Royal Commission on Health Services recommended public coverage for a broad range of services including pharmacare and home care. The Canadian Medical Association opposed the *Canada Health Act* and even Prime Minister Pearson's minority Liberal government was split ideologically. The watered down *Act* included no coverage beyond physicians' services.

The *Canada Health Act* does mention extended health care services which it defines as "nursing home intermediate care, adult residential care, home care, and ambulatory health care services." In the 1980s, there were small grants given to the provinces to develop their continuing care systems. However, the *Act's* main focus is hospital and physicians' services, and this reinforces the perspective that continuing care is an optional extra for the provinces.

On a positive note, the federal government, the provinces, and the territories included a paragraph on home care as part of the 2004 *Health Accord.* Even so, the limited "guarantee" of first-dollar coverage for palliative care and two weeks of post-hospital care has been as inconsistently implemented as the other key provisions of the agreement.

Since the 1990s, provincial governments have off-loaded their financial responsibilities by ensuring that they do not pay for services that aren't explicitly included in the *Canada Health Act*. As noted by British Columbia's Marcia Carr, that province is now charging patients for 6-8 week courses of rehabilitation after acute care.

There has also been a significant decrease in the availability of publicly paid continuing care institutional beds. By 2008, there were 15% fewer funded public institutional continuing care beds for Canadians over 75, and 25% fewer for those over 85.

For-profit "independent living" institutions and unregulated "retirement homes" have jumped into this vacuum. These facilities offer services such as bathing and personal care off an *à la carte* menu. Usually residents need few services upon entry, but as their needs increase, the costs can rise to thousands of dollars per month. Residents empty their savings while they wait for a publicly funded continuing care bed.

There is no doubt that some of the money used for institutional long-term care could be better spent. Although all Canadian hospitals are non-profit, over one third of continuing care institutional beds are located in for-profit facilities. Research in several provinces shows that for-profit facilities tend to have fewer and less well-trained staff and provide poorer quality of care.

This policy of retrenchment of publicly funded continuing care services is short-sighted. It compromises the integrity of the public system because continuing care services reduce the demand for hospital care. Ontario Ombudsman André Marin noted in a recent report that up to 20% of patients in hospital beds actually require continuing care either in a facility or the community. And, many of these hospital admissions could have been prevented if the patient had been receiving continuing care prior to the hospitalization.

In the late 1990s, some health regions in BC reduced coverage for so-called supportive home care services such as housekeeping. Other regions didn't make these cutbacks. Victoria-based researcher Dr. Marcus Hollander took advantage of this natural experiment to compare the costs of those who lost their services to those who retained them. In the first year there was little difference, but by the third year the elderly who lost their supportive services used 50% more health care than those who retained them. The biggest costs were related to hospital care.

Denmark — a country where health care system is almost entirely publicly run and financed — provides a national level example of how to deal with an aging population. In 1987, Denmark made a policy decision to provide the same benefits for drugs, supplies, and durable medical equipment to elderly living in the community as those in institutions. The key to receiving services was not the location of services provided, but rather the patient's assessed need for care. At the same time, Denmark greatly accelerated the construction of supportive housing. Supportive care, personal care, and other publicly financed services are available on an as-needed basis.

In 1998, Denmark developed a country-wide program of regular nursing visits to those over 75 years of age. The nurses ensure that elders who are beginning to fail are identified early, and services are provided before they enter a crisis situation. As a result, Denmark's hospital system is not gridlocked, and despite Denmark having an older population than Canada, the Danes spend less on health care than we do in Canada.

Continuing care is far from a frill. Successful health systems ensure that continuing care services are publicly covered and integrated with other health and social services.

To move forward in Canada, we need to focus on better integration at three levels. First, we need the federal government and the provinces to integrate their policies on continuing care. We need to legally regard continuing care like necessary medical and hospital care. We should provide it without charge to all Canadians who need it. As in Denmark, people should have coverage for their services (like drugs, medical supplies, etc.) according to their needs, not according to their place of residence.

Second, federal and provincial governments need to better integrate their planning for an aging population across the continuum of care. Currently we have the siloed perspectives of three layers of governments and different government departments such as health care, social services, housing, etc. Status Aboriginals have a fourth layer of government.

Successful continuing care requires reform of our pension programs, the construction of supportive housing, and initiatives to make transportation for the elderly and disabled more user-friendly. All of these initiatives require more effective coordination of social policy.

Finally, provincial and territorial governments need to better integrate their health care systems. We need to refer emergency room patients directly to continuing care without having to endure an unnecessary and potentially dangerous hospitalization.

As in Denmark, we should provide continuing care as soon as it is needed by reaching out to seniors before they are in crisis.

We need to ensure that we have the skilled staff necessary to provide continuing care. In some provinces those who work in continuing care are well-trained and fairly compensated. But too much continuing care is provided by poorly trained and often unregulated staff who are not making a living wage.

Too often Canadians in need have to rely on care provided by unpaid family members and friends. Too often these care providers sacrifice their own lives, careers, and pensions to deliver dignity to their loved ones. We cannot maintain the integrity of the continuing care system without well-trained, fairly paid staff delivering services that are accessible to all Canadians in a timely fashion.

Athletes perpetually train for the next Olympics. Today, medicare advocates should be hard in training for the next federal-provincial-territorial *Accord* in 2014. The 2004 agreement did allow the Martin government to say it was back in the health care game after nearly twenty years of federal cuts to transfer payments.

However, the agreement which was supposed to heal health care for a generation fell apart in a fruit fly's lifetime. Within weeks, some provinces were saying they were unhappy with key provisions and threatening to go private. The need for federal leadership in initiating a national discussion on continuing care cannot be understated.

The elephant in the room as we discuss social policy is that Canadian governments have slashed their own revenue base. From 2000 to 2008, taxes were cut by 5.3% of GDP, which amounts to roughly $85 billion in foregone annual revenue. If governments had kept just half of these revenues, there would be no government deficits in 2011/2012. Canadians want a universal continuing care program as well as pharmacare, universal early childhood education, and a national housing program.

The moral test of any society is how it treats its most vulnerable members. Alberta consumer activist Wendy Armstrong reminds us that the key value underpinning medicare is that we should all share the burden of care when someone attains a certain level of need. Canadians believe in the values for fairness and social justice. We need to ensure that our politicians do too.

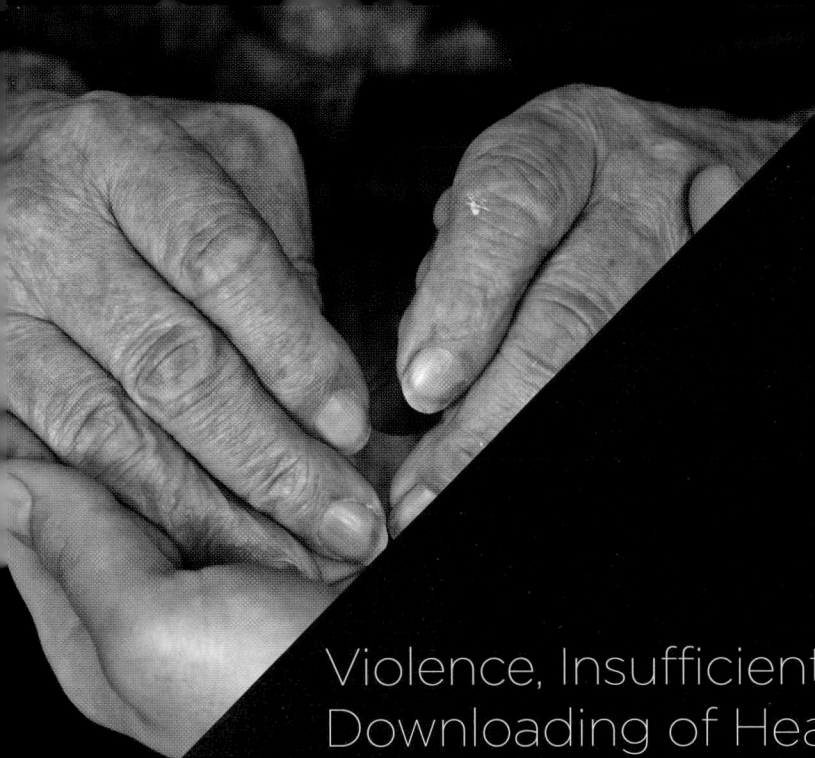

Violence, Insufficient Care, and Downloading of Heavy Care Patients: An Evaluation of Increasing Need and Inadequate Standards in Ontario's Nursing Homes

"There is a need to redirect funding and policy attention to quality of care issues. Care workers regularly report to us that they are unable to meet health and safety and professional standards at current staffing levels. Residents report unsafe or inadequate living conditions, lack of palliative care, and deeply disturbing concerns about quality of care, outcomes and quality of life. Families echo stories of a culture of fear, guilt, stress, and inadequate care."

Ontario Health Coalition. (2008). *Violence, Insufficient Care, and Downloading of Heavy Care Patients: An evaluation of increasing need and inadequate standards in Ontario's nursing homes.* Ottawa: Author. Retrieved from:
http://www.web.net/ohc/LongTermCare.htm#LReports